Understanding Nutrition and Metabolism

Understanding Nutrition and Metabolism

Elsa Holt

Callisto Reference

www.callistoreference.com

Callisto Reference,
118-35 Queens Blvd., Suite 400,
Forest Hills, NY 11375, USA

Visit us on the World Wide Web at:
www.callistoreference.com

ISBN: 978-1-64116-420-7 (Hardback)

Printed in China.

Cataloging-in-Publication Data

Understanding nutrition and metabolism / Elsa Holt.
p. cm.
Includes bibliographical references and index.
ISBN 978-1-64116-420-7
1. Nutrition. 2. Metabolism. 3. Health. I. Holt, Elsa.

QP141 .N88 2020
613.2--dc23

Table of Contents

Preface

The purpose of this book is to help students understand the fundamental concepts of this discipline. It is designed to motivate students to learn and prosper. I am grateful for the support of my colleagues. I would also like to acknowledge the encouragement of my family.

The science that interprets the interaction of nutrients and other substances found in food and their role in the health of an organism is known as nutrition. It also deals with the maintenance, growth, reproduction and disease in organisms with respect to nutrients. Some of the processes which are studied under nutrition are food intake, assimilation, biosynthesis, catabolism and excretion. Proper nutrition is essential to avoid deficiency-related diseases like anemia, blindness, scurvy, stillbirth, preterm birth and cretinism. Metabolism is a group of life-sustaining chemical reactions in organisms. It helps in the conversion of food to energy for running cellular processes. It also converts the food to building blocks for proteins, nucleic acids, lipids and carbohydrates. Proper nutrition is essential for metabolism since metabolic pathways depend upon nutrients which they breakdown to produce energy. This book is a compilation of chapters that discuss the most vital concepts in the fields of nutrition and metabolism. The topics covered herein deal with the core aspects of these areas. This book will provide comprehensive knowledge to the readers.

A foreword for all the chapters is provided below:

Chapter – Understanding Nutrition

Nutrition is a science which studies the interaction of nutrients and other constituents of food with respect to growth, health, reproduction and disease of an organism. One of the many branches of nutrition is sports nutrition, which seeks to improve athletic performance through nutrition and diet. This is an introductory chapter which is going to give a brief introduction about these aspects of nutrition.

Chapter – Metabolism and Metabolic Pathways

The set of chemical reactions which are vital for the sustenance of life is known as metabolism. The different metabolic reactions are organized into metabolic pathways, where a chemical is transformed into another chemical through a series of steps. This chapter has been carefully written to provide an easy understanding of the varied facets of metabolism such as microbial metabolism and ATP in metabolism.

Chapter – Macronutrients and their Metabolism

Some of the major macronutrients which are present in the body are carbohydrates, fats and proteins. Their metabolism refers to the various biochemical processes due to which the formation, breakdown and interconversion of these macronutrients takes place within living organisms. This chapter discusses in detail the processes related to the metabolism of these macronutrients.

Chapter – Micronutrients: Vitamins and Minerals

The micronutrients within the body are divided into two broad categories, vitamins and minerals. Some of the different vitamins are vitamin A, B, C, D, E and K. There are a number of minerals which are vital for metabolism such as manganese, calcium and phosphorus. This chapter has been carefully written to provide an easy understanding of these varied micronutrients.

Chapter – Role of Enzymes in Metabolism

Enzymes are large molecular biological catalysts which are responsible for increasing the rate of chemical reactions. They play a vital role in the metabolic processes by increasing the reaction rates without altering the chemical equilibrium which exists between the products and reactants. The chapter closely examines these key roles of enzymes in metabolism to provide an extensive understanding of the subject.

Elsa Holt

1
Understanding Nutrition

Nutrition is a science which studies the interaction of nutrients and other constituents of food with respect to growth, health, reproduction and disease of an organism. One of the many branches of nutrition is sports nutrition, which seeks to improve athletic performance through nutrition and diet. This is an introductory chapter which is going to give a brief introduction about these aspects of nutrition.

Nutrition is defined as the processes by which living organisms takes in and utilises food substances. Essential nutrients include protein, carbohydrate, fat, vitamins, minerals and electrolytes. Normally, 85% of daily energy use is from fat and carbohydrates and 15% from protein. In humans, nutrition is mainly achieved through the process of putting foods into our mouths, chewing and swallowing it. The required amounts of the essential nutrients differ by age and the state of the body, for example: physical activity, diseases present (e.g. prostate cancer, breast cancer or weakened bones – known as osteoporosis), medications, pregnancy and lactation.

Importance of Nutrition

Nutrition is essential for growth and development, health and wellbeing. Eating a healthy diet contributes to preventing future illness and improving quality and length of life. Your nutritional status is the state of your health as determined by what you eat. There are several ways of assessing nutritional status, including anthropometric (i.e. physical body measurement), food intake and biochemical measurement.

Human Nutrition

Human nutrition is the process by which substances in food are transformed into body tissues and provide energy for the full range of physical and mental activities that make up human life.

The study of human nutrition is interdisciplinary in character, involving not only physiology, biochemistry, and molecular biology but also fields such as psychology and anthropology, which explore the influence of attitudes, beliefs, preferences, and cultural traditions on food choices. Human nutrition further touches on economics and political science as the world community recognizes and responds to the suffering and death caused by malnutrition. The ultimate goal of nutritional science is to promote optimal health and reduce the risk of chronic diseases such as cardiovascular disease and cancer as well as to prevent classic nutritional deficiency diseases such as kwashiorkor and pellagra.

Utilization of Food by the Body

Calories and Kilocalories: Energy Supply

The human body can be thought of as an engine that releases the energy present in the foods that it digests. This energy is utilized partly for the mechanical work performed by the muscles and in the secretory processes and partly for the work necessary to maintain the body's structure and functions. The performance of work is associated with the production of heat; heat loss is controlled so as to keep body temperature within a narrow range. Unlike other engines, however, the human body is continually breaking down (catabolizing) and building up (anabolizing) its component parts. Foods supply nutrients essential to the manufacture of the new material and provide energy needed for the chemical reactions involved.

Carbohydrate, fat, and protein are, to a large extent, interchangeable as sources of energy. Typically, the energy provided by food is measured in kilocalories, or Calories. One kilocalorie is equal to 1,000 gram-calories (or small calories), a measure of heat energy. However, in common parlance, kilocalories are referred to as "calories." In other words, a 2,000-calorie diet actually has 2,000 kilocalories of potential energy. One kilocalorie is the amount of heat energy required to raise one kilogram of water from 14.5 to 15.5 °C at one atmosphere of pressure. Another unit of energy widely used is the joule, which measures energy in terms of mechanical work. One joule is the energy expended when one kilogram is moved a distance of one metre by a force of one newton. The relatively higher levels of energy in human nutrition are more likely to be measured in kilojoules (1 kilojoule = 10^3 joules) or megajoules (1 megajoule = 10^6 joules). One kilocalorie is equivalent to 4.184 kilojoules.

The energy present in food can be determined directly by measuring the output of heat when the food is burned (oxidized) in a bomb calorimeter. However, the human body is not as efficient as a calorimeter, and some potential energy is lost during digestion and metabolism. Corrected physiological values for the heats of combustion of the three energy-yielding nutrients, rounded to whole numbers, are as follows: carbohydrate, 4 kilocalories (17 kilojoules) per gram; protein, 4 kilocalories (17 kilojoules) per gram; and fat, 9 kilocalories (38 kilojoules) per gram. Beverage alcohol (ethyl alcohol) also yields energy—7 kilocalories (29 kilojoules) per gram—although it is not essential in the diet. Vitamins, minerals, water, and other food constituents have no energy value, although many of them participate in energy-releasing processes in the body.

The energy provided by a well-digested food can be estimated if the gram amounts of energy-yielding substances (non-fibre carbohydrate, fat, protein, and alcohol) in that food are known. For example, a slice of white bread containing 12 grams of carbohydrate, 2 grams of protein, and 1 gram of fat supplies 67 kilocalories (280 kilojoules) of energy. Food composition tables and food labels provide useful data for evaluating energy and nutrient intake of an individual diet. Most foods provide a mixture of energy-supplying nutrients, along with vitamins, minerals, water, and other substances. Two notable exceptions are table sugar and vegetable oil, which are virtually pure carbohydrate (sucrose) and fat, respectively.

Throughout most of the world, protein supplies between 8 and 16 percent of the energy in the diet, although there are wide variations in the proportions of fat and carbohydrate in different populations. In more prosperous communities about 12 to 15 percent of energy is typically derived from protein, 30 to 40 percent from fat, and 50 to 60 percent from carbohydrate. On the other hand, in many poorer agricultural societies, where cereals comprise the bulk of the diet, carbohydrate provides an even larger percentage of energy, with protein and fat providing less. The human body is remarkably adaptable and can survive, and even thrive, on widely divergent diets. However, different dietary patterns are associated with particular health consequences.

BMR and REE: Energy Balance

Energy is needed not only when a person is physically active but even when the body is lying motionless. Depending on an individual's level of physical activity, between 50 and 80 percent of the energy expended each day is devoted to basic metabolic processes (basal metabolism), which enable the body to stay warm, breathe, pump blood, and conduct numerous physiological and biosynthetic activities, including synthesis of new tissue in growing children and in pregnant and lactating women. Digestion and subsequent processing of food by the body also uses energy and produces heat. This phenomenon, known as the thermic effect of food (or diet-induced thermogenesis), accounts for about 10 percent of daily energy expenditure, varying somewhat with the composition of the diet and prior dietary practices. Adaptive thermogenesis, another small but important component of energy expenditure, reflects alterations in metabolism due to changes in ambient temperature, hormone production, emotional stress, or other factors. Finally, the most variable component in energy expenditure is physical activity, which includes exercise and other voluntary activities as well as involuntary activities such as fidgeting, shivering, and maintaining posture. Physical activity accounts for 20 to 40 percent of the total energy expenditure, even less in a very sedentary person and more in someone who is extremely active.

Basal or resting energy expenditure is correlated primarily with lean body mass (fat-free mass and essential fat, excluding storage fat), which is the metabolically active tissue in the body. At rest, organs such as the liver, brain, heart, and kidney have the highest metabolic activity and, therefore, the highest need for energy, while muscle and bone require less energy, and body fat even less. Besides body composition, other factors affecting basal metabolism include age, sex, body temperature, and thyroid hormone levels.

The basal metabolic rate (BMR), a precisely defined measure of the energy expenditure necessary to support life, is determined under controlled and standardized conditions—shortly after awakening in the morning, at least 12 hours after the last meal, and with a comfortable room temperature. Because of practical considerations, the BMR is rarely measured; the resting energy expenditure (REE) is determined under less stringent conditions, with the individual resting comfortably about 2 to 4 hours after a meal. In practice, the BMR and REE differ by no more than 10 percent—the REE is usually slightly higher—and the terms are used interchangeably.

Energy expenditure can be assessed by direct calorimetry, or measurement of heat dissipated from the body, which employs apparatuses such as water-cooled garments or insulated chambers large enough to accommodate a person. However, energy expenditure is usually measured by the less cumbersome techniques of indirect calorimetry, in which heat produced by the body is calculated from measurements of oxygen inhaled, carbon dioxide exhaled, and urinary nitrogen excreted. The BMR (in kilocalories per day) can be roughly estimated using the following formula: $BMR = 70 \times (\text{body weight in kilograms})^{3/4}$.

The energy costs of various activities have been measured. While resting may require as little as 1 kilocalorie per minute, strenuous work may demand 10 times that much. Mental activity, though it may seem taxing, has no appreciable effect on energy requirement. A 70-kg (154-pound) man, whose REE over the course of a day might be 1,750 kilocalories, could expend a total of 2,400 kilocalories on a very sedentary day and up to 4,000 kilocalories on a very active day. A 55-kg (121-pound) woman, whose daily resting energy expenditure might be 1,350 kilocalories, could use from 1,850 to more than 3,000 total kilocalories, depending on level of activity.

Approximate energy expenditure for activity levels		
Activity category	Energy as multiple of resting energy expenditure (ree)	Kilocalories per minute
Resting (sleeping, reclining)	REE × 1.0	1–1.2
Very light (driving, typing, cooking)	REE × 1.5	up to 2.5
Light (walking on a level surface at 4 to 5 km/hr [2.5 To 3 mph], golf, table tennis)	REE × 2.5	2.5–4.9
Moderate (walking 5.5 To 6.5 Km/hr [3.5 To 4 mph], carrying a load, cycling, tennis, skiing, dancing)	REE × 5.0	5.0–7.4
Heavy (walking uphill with a load, basketball, climbing, football, soccer)	REE × 7.0	7.5–12.0

The law of conservation of energy applies: If one takes in more energy than is expended, over time one will gain weight; insufficient energy intake results in weight loss, as the body taps its energy stores to provide for immediate needs. Excess food energy is stored in small amounts as glycogen, a short-term storage form of carbohydrate in muscle and liver, and as fat, the body's main energy reserve found in adipose tissue. Adipose tissue is mostly fat (about 87 percent), but it also contains some protein and water. In order to lose 454 grams (one pound) of adipose tissue, an energy deficit of about 3,500 kilocalories (14.6 megajoules) is required.

Body Mass, Body Fat and Body Water

The human body consists of materials similar to those found in foods; however, the relative proportions differ, according to genetic dictates as well as to the unique life experience of the individual. The body of a healthy lean man is composed of roughly 62 percent water, 16 percent fat, 16 percent protein, 6 percent minerals, and less than 1 percent carbohydrate, along with very small amounts of vitamins and other miscellaneous substances. Females usually carry more fat (about 22 percent in a healthy lean woman) and slightly less of the other components than do males of comparable weight.

The body's different compartments—lean body mass, body fat, and body water—are constantly adjusting to changes in the internal and external environment so that a state of dynamic equilibrium (homeostasis) is maintained. Tissues in the body are continuously being broken down (catabolism) and built up (anabolism) at varying rates. For example, the epithelial cells lining the digestive tract are replaced at a dizzying speed of every three or four days, while the life span of red blood cells is 120 days, and connective tissue is renewed over the course of several years.

Although estimates of the percentage of body fat can be made by direct inspection, this approach is imprecise. Body fat can be measured indirectly using fairly precise but costly methods, such as underwater weighing, total body potassium counting, and dual-energy X-ray absorptiometry (DXA). However, more practical, albeit less accurate, methods are often used, such as anthropometry, in which subcutaneous fat at various sites is measured using skinfold calipers; bioelectrical impedance, in which resistance to a low-intensity electrical current is used to estimate body fat; and near infrared interactance, in which an infrared light aimed at the biceps is used to assess fat and protein interaction. Direct measurement of the body's various compartments can only be performed on cadavers.

The composition of the body tends to change in somewhat predictable ways over the course of a lifetime—during the growing years, in pregnancy and lactation, and as one ages—with corresponding changes in nutrient needs during different phases of the life cycle. Regular physical exercise can help attenuate the age-related loss of lean tissue and increase in body fat.

Essential Nutrient Requirements

Nutrients can be described as the chemical components of food and can be classified into six broad groups: carbohydrates, proteins, fats, vitamins, minerals and water. Water is not technically a nutrient, but it is essential for the utilisation of nutrients. Nutrients perform various functions in our bodies, including energy provision and maintaining vital processes such as digestion, breathing, growth and development.

Energy Balance

Your energy requirement depends on your age, size and activity level. If your energy intake equals the amount of energy you expend, then you are in energy balance. If your intake exceeds your expenditure, the excess energy is converted to body fat and you gain weight. On the other hand, if your intake is less than your expenditure, your body uses up fat stores and you lose weight. Therefore, for weight to remain stable, the total amount of calories that are consumed must not exceed the total that is used up through metabolic processes (e.g. exercising, sweating, breathing). Energy intake must match energy output. The average energy intake is about 2800 kcal/day for men and 1800 kcal/day for women, although this varies with body size and activity level.

Carbohydrates

Carbohydrates can be classified as monosaccharide (e.g. glucose, fructose, galactose), disaccharide (e.g. sucrose, lactose, maltose) and polysaccharide (e.g. starch, fibre). Carbohydrates must be reduced to the simplest form of glucose (through digestion) before your body can make use of them. Carbohydrates should make up at least 55% of your total energy intake. The brain is a special part of the body that depends primarily on glucose for its energy and requires about 100 g/day of glucose for fuel. In some situations, the body can compensate for decreased levels of carbohydrates by using alternative energy pathways such as burning fatty acids.

Protein

Protein is important for the production, maintenance and repair of tissues in the body. When energy intake is insufficient, protein intake must be raised. This is because ingested proteins are preferentially directed towards glucose (sugar) synthesis and oxidation. The tissues and organs in the body are made up of protein and protein compounds. Enzymes (biological catalysts), antibodies and hormones also consist of protein. The building blocks of protein are called amino acids. The body can make all of the 20 amino acids except eight, which are termed essential amino acids. These are isoleucine, leucine, lysine, methionine, phenylalanine, threonine, tryptophan and valine. Histidine is essential only for infants. The number and nature of amino acids present in a particular protein determines that protein's characteristics.

For adults, the recommended dietary allowance of protein is about 0.75 g/kg body weight per day. Animal products tend to have the highest amount of proteins, followed by legumes (beans), cereals (rice, wheat, corn) and roots. Animal protein (from meat, eggs, fish, milk) contains all the essential amino acids and is normally referred to as 'complete' or 'high biological value' protein. Protein derived from plants lack one or two essential amino acids. However, a good combination of plant-based protein can be of equal value to animal protein. For example, legumes lack methionine but have adequate amounts of lysine. Cereals, on the other hand, lack lysine but have a lot of methionine. Therefore, a mixture of rice and beans will supply all the essential amino acids.

Excess protein cannot be stored in the body, so we need to consume protein daily. Consuming too much protein is not recommended because it promotes increased calcium excretion through urine, which increases the risk of developing osteoporosis. Additionally, too much protein intake may lead to a greater concentration of the amino acid homocysteine in the blood, and the subsequent conversion to thiolactone. Thiolactone is associated with increased levels of atherosclerosis and endothelial damage.

Fats and Oils

Most of the fats we consume occur in foods as triglycerides. A triglyceride is comprised of three fatty acid molecules attached to a glycerol molecule. Fatty acids are made up of carbon and hydrogen atoms and can be either saturated or unsaturated. Saturated fatty acids (SFA) have the maximum number of hydrogen atoms attached to the carbon chain, while unsaturated fatty acids have less than the required hydrogen atoms. For example, monounsaturated fatty acids (e.g. oleic acid) have two hydrogen atoms missing. Monounsaturated fats are found mainly in nuts, avocados, olive oil, canola oil, grapeseed oil, peanut oil, flaxseed oil, sesame oil, corn oil, safflower oil, sunflower oil, etc.

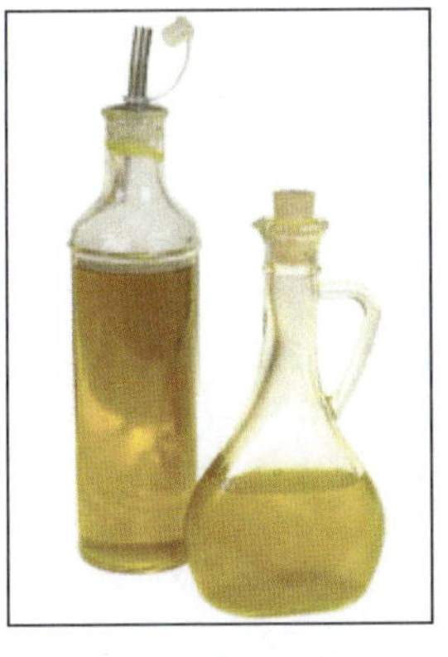

Polyunsaturated fatty acids (PUFA) have more than two hydrogen atoms missing (e.g. linoleic acid and linolenic acid). Linoleic and linolenic acids are regarded as essential fatty acids (EFAs) because the body cannot make them. There are two categories of EFAs: omega-3 and omega-6. The number that comes after "omega-" represents the position of the first double bond, counting from the terminal methyl group on the molecule. Omega-3 fatty acids are derived from linolenic acid and omega-6 from linoleic acid. Alpha linolenic acid (ALA) is converted into eicosapentaenoic acid (EPA), and later into docosahexaenoic acid (DHA) in the body. Sources of omega-3 fats include salmon, mackerel, sardines, anchovies, tuna, flaxseed oil, walnuts, etc. Sources of omega-6 fats include palm oil, soybean oil, canola oil, sunflower oil, nuts, etc. Evidence from research indicates that omega-3 fatty acids reduce inflammation and help prevent certain chronic diseases such as heart disease and arthritis. Omega-3 fatty acids are highly concentrated in the brain and appear to be crucial to brain function as well as normal growth and development. Infants who do not get enough omega-3 fatty acids from their mothers during pregnancy are at risk of mental impairment.

Generally, saturated fatty acids raise blood cholesterol levels, whereas unsaturated fatty acids lower them. Saturated fats are found in foods such as butter, meat and dairy fats. Trans fats are artificially created during food processing. In the body, trans fats act in a similar way to saturated fats and may raise cholesterol levels. These fats are considered to be harmful to your health. Trans fats are found mainly in deep-fried fast foods and processed foods made with margarine.

Fats are a concentrated and rich source of energy. It is recommended that your total fat intake is no more than 30% of your energy (calorie/kilojoule) intake. Polyunsaturated fat should be less than 10% of energy, and saturated fat and trans fat together should be less than 10%. The rest of your fat intake should consist of monounsaturated fat.

Vitamins

Vitamins constitute a group of nutrients that are needed in small quantities. Like amino and fatty acids, most vitamins cannot be made in the body and must be obtained from dietary sources. Only vitamin D can be manufactured by the body. Essential vitamins are grouped into two families: water soluble and fat soluble. Water soluble vitamins can dissolve in water (thiamine, riboflavin, niacin, vitamin C, folic acid). These cannot be stored by the body and need to be consumed every day. Fat soluble vitamins can dissolve in a fat medium (vitamins A, D, E, K). These are taken into our bodies when we consume fat-containing foods. Vitamins are needed for various reasons, including the formation of hormones and blood cells. They generally act as coenzymes. An inadequate supply of vitamins in our diet leads to the development of diseases.

- Vitamin A: Derived from carotene, vitamin A affects vision, reproduction, and the formation and maintenance of skin, mucous membranes, bones and teeth. Deficiency results in night blindness (difficulty in adapting to darkness). The body obtains vitamin A from either carotene (vitamin A precursor) or by absorbing ready-made vitamin A from plant-eating organisms. Carotene is found in dark green leafy vegetables and yellow-orange fruit/vegetables. Pre formed vitamin A is found in milk, butter, cheese, egg yolk, liver, and fish-liver oil.

- Vitamin B complex: The vitamin B complex is a mixture of eight essential vitamins necessary to enhance immune and nervous system function, and promote cell growth and division. Pregnant or lactating women, alcoholics and the elderly are more likely to suffer from vitamin B deficiency.
- Vitamin B1 (thiamine): Thiamine, or vitamin B1, acts as a catalyst in carbohydrate metabolism. Thiamine deficiency causes beriberi, a vitamin deficiency disorder characterised by muscular weakness, swelling of the heart and leg cramps. In severe cases, beriberi may lead to heart failure and death. The richest dietary sources of thiamine are organ meats (liver, heart, and kidney), brewer's yeast, lean meats, eggs, leafy green vegetables, whole or enriched cereals, wheat germ, berries, nuts, and legumes.
- Vitamin B2 (riboflavin): Riboflavin, or vitamin B2, acts as a coenzyme in the metabolism of carbohydrates, fats, and respiratory proteins. The best sources of riboflavin are liver, milk, meat, dark green vegetables, whole grain and enriched cereals, pasta, bread and mushrooms.
- Vitamin B6 (pyroxidine): Pyridoxine, or vitamin B6, is necessary for the absorption and metabolism of amino acids. It also plays a role in the body's use of fats and in the formation of red blood cells. The best sources of pyridoxine are whole grains, cereals, bread, liver, avocados, spinach, green beans and bananas.
- Folic acid (vitamin B9 or folacin): Folic acid is a coenzyme needed for forming body protein and haemoglobin. Folic acid deficiency is associated with neural tube defects. Dietary sources are organ meats, leafy green vegetables, legumes, nuts, whole grains and brewer's yeast. Folic acid is lost in foods stored at room temperature and during cooking.

Minerals

Minerals are essential, acting as cofactors of enzymes (i.e. enzymes would not exist or function without minerals). Some of the minerals necessary for health are:

- Calcium: Calcium is a very important mineral in the diet, especially for women at menopause. The major function of calcium is to build and help maintain strong bones. It can stop the onset of osteoporosis and reduce bone loss and fragility. It is involved in blood clotting. Calcium deficiency can develop when there is a lack of vitamin D.
- Iron: Iron in food exists as haem and non-haem iron. Haem iron, found in red meat, is relatively well (20–30%) absorbed. Non-haem iron, found mostly in cereals, pulses, certain vegetables (e.g. spinach) and eggs, is generally less well absorbed. Non-haem iron absorption depends on other factors in the diet. For example, vitamin C and animal protein enhance non-haem iron absorption, while tea, coffee and phytates inhibit it.

- Zinc: Zinc represents only 0.003% of the human body, but is essential for synthesising protein, DNA and RNA. It is required for growth in all stages of life. Sources include meats, oysters and other seafood, milk, and egg yolk.

Food Groups

The following nine food groups reflect foods with generally similar nutritional characteristics: (1) cereals, (2) starchy roots, (3) legumes, (4) vegetables and fruits, (5) sugars, preserves, and syrups, (6) meat, fish, and eggs, (7) milk and milk products, (8) fats and oils, and (9) beverages.

Cereals

The cereals are all grasses that have been bred over millennia to bear large seeds (i.e., grain). The most important cereals for human consumption are rice, wheat, and corn (maize). Others include barley, oats, and millet. The carbohydrate-rich cereals compare favourably with the protein-rich foods in energy value; in addition, the cost of production (per calorie) of cereals is less than that of almost all other foods and they can be stored dry for many years. Therefore, most of the world's diets are arranged to meet main calorie requirements from the cheaper carbohydrate foods. The major component of all grains is starch. Cereals contain little fat, with oats having an exceptional 9 percent. The amount of protein in cereals ranges from 6 to 16 percent but does not have as high a nutritive value as that of many animal foods because of the low lysine content.

Controversy exists as to the relative merits of white bread and bread made from whole wheat flour. White flour consists of about 72 percent of the grain but contains little of the germ (embryo) and of the outer coverings (bran). Since the B vitamins are concentrated mainly in the scutellum (covering of the germ), and to a lesser extent in the bran, the vitamin B content of white flour, unless artificially enriched, is less than that of brown flour. Dietary fibre is located mostly in the bran, so that white flour contains only about one-third of that in whole wheat flour. White flour is compulsorily enriched with synthetic vitamins in a number of countries, including the United States and the United Kingdom, so that the vitamin content is similar to that of the darker flours. White flour, of course, still lacks fibre and any yet unidentified beneficial factors that may be present in the outer layers of the wheat.

B vitamins are also lost when brown rice is polished to yield white rice. People living on white rice and little else are at risk for developing the disease beriberi, which is caused by a deficiency of thiamin (vitamin B_1). Beriberi was formerly common in poor Asian communities in which a large proportion of the diet consisted of polished rice. The disease has almost completely disappeared from Asia with the advent of greater availability of other foods and, in some areas, fortification of the rice with thiamin.

Yellow corn differs from other cereals in that it contains carotenoids with vitamin A activity. (Another exception is a genetically modified so-called golden rice, which contains carotene, the precursor for vitamin A.) Corn is also lower in the amino acid tryptophan than other cereals. The niacin in corn is in a bound form that cannot be digested or absorbed by humans unless pretreated with lime (calcium hydroxide) or unless immature grains are eaten at the so-called milky stage (usually as sweet corn). Niacin is also formed in the body as a metabolite of the amino acid tryptophan, but this alternative source is not available when the tryptophan content is too low.

Starchy Roots

Starchy roots consumed in large quantities include potatoes, sweet potatoes, yams, taro, and cassava. Their nutritive value in general resembles that of cereals. The potato, however, provides some protein (2 percent) and also contains vitamin C. The yellow-fleshed varieties of sweet potato contain the pigment beta-carotene, convertible in the body into vitamin A. Cassava is extremely low in protein, and most varieties contain cyanide-forming compounds that make them toxic unless processed correctly.

Legumes

Beans and peas are the seeds of leguminous crops that are able to utilize atmospheric nitrogen via parasitic microorganisms attached to their roots. Legumes contain at least 20 percent protein, and they are a good source of most of the B vitamins and of iron. Like cereals, most legumes are low in fat; an important exception is the soybean (17 percent), a major commercial source of edible oil. Tofu, or bean curd, is made from soybeans and is an important source of protein in China, Japan, Korea, and Southeast Asia. Peanuts (groundnuts) are also the seeds of a leguminous plant, although they ripen underground; much of the crop is processed for its oil.

Vegetables and Fruits

Vegetables and fruits have similar nutritive properties. Because 70 percent or more of their weight is water, they provide comparatively little energy or protein, but many contain vitamin C and carotene. However, cooked vegetables are an uncertain source of vitamin C, as this vitamin is easily destroyed by heat. The dark-green leafy vegetables are particularly good sources of vitamin A activity. Vegetables also provide calcium and iron but often in a form that is poorly absorbed. The more typical fruits, such as apples, oranges, and berries, are rich in sugar. Bananas are a good source of potassium. Vegetables and fruits also contain fibre, which adds bulk to the intestinal content and is useful in preventing constipation.

Botanically, nuts are actually a kind of fruit, but they are quite different in character with their hard shell and high fat content. The coconut, for example, contains some 60 percent fat when dried. Olives are another fruit rich in fat and are traditionally grown for their oil.

Sugars, Preserves and Syrups

One characteristic of diets of affluent societies is their high content of sugar. This is due in part to sugar added at the table or as an ingredient in candy, preserves, and sweetened colas or other beverages. There are also naturally occurring sugars in foods (lactose in milk and fructose, glucose, and sucrose in fruits and some vegetables). Sugar, however, contains no protein, minerals, or vitamins and thus has been called the source of "empty calories".

Because sugar adsorbs water and prevents the growth of microorganisms, it is an excellent preservative. Making jam or marmalade is a way of preserving fruit, but most of the vitamin C is destroyed, and the products contain up to 70 percent sugar. Honey and natural syrups (e.g., maple syrup) are composed of more than 75 percent sugar.

Meat, Fish and Eggs

Generally meats consist of about 20 percent protein, 20 percent fat, and 60 percent water. The amount of fat present in a particular portion of meat varies greatly, not only with the kind of meat but also with the quality; the "energy value" varies in direct proportion with the fat content. Meat is valuable for its protein, which is of high biological value. Pork is an excellent source of thiamin. Meat is also a good source of niacin, vitamin B_{12}, vitamin B_6, and the mineral nutrients iron, zinc, phosphorus, potassium, and magnesium. Liver is the storage organ for, and is very rich in, vitamin A, riboflavin, and folic acid. In many cultures the organs (offal) of animals—including the kidneys, the heart, the tongue, and the liver—are considered delicacies. Liver is a particularly rich source of many vitamins.

The muscular tissue of fishes consists of 13 to 20 percent protein, fat ranging from less than 1 to more than 20 percent, and 60 to 82 percent water that varies inversely with fat content. Many species of fish, such as cod and haddock, concentrate fat in the liver and as a result have extremely lean muscles. The tissues of other fish, such as salmon and herring, may contain 15 percent fat or more. However, fish oil, unlike the fat in land animals, is rich in essential long-chain fatty acids, particularly eicosapentaenoic acid.

The egg has a deservedly high reputation as a food. Its white contains protein, and its yolk is rich in both protein and vitamin A. An egg also provides calcium and iron. Egg yolk, however, has a high cholesterol content.

Milk and Milk Products

The milk of each species of animal is a complete food for its young. Moreover, one pint of cow's milk contributes about 90 percent of the calcium, 30 to 40 percent of the riboflavin, 25 to 30 percent of the protein, 10 to 20 percent of the calories and vitamins A and B, and up to 10 percent of the iron and vitamin D needed by a human adult.

Human breast milk is the perfect food for infants, provided it comes from a healthy, well-nourished mother and the infant is full-term. Breast milk contains important antibodies, white blood cells, and nutrients. In communities where hygiene is poor, breast-fed babies have fewer infections than formula-fed babies. In the past, infants who could not be breast-fed were given cow's milk that was partially "humanized" with the addition of water and a small amount of sugar or wheat flour. However, this was far from an ideal substitute for breast milk, being lower in iron and containing undenatured proteins that could produce allergic reactions with bleeding into the gut and, in some cases, eczema.

Lactose, the characteristic sugar of milk, is a disaccharide made of the monosaccharides glucose and galactose. Some adults can break down the lactose of large quantities of milk into galactose and glucose, but others have an inherited lactose intolerance as a result of the lactase enzyme no longer being secreted into the gut after the age of weaning. As a result, unabsorbed lactose is fermented by bacteria and produces bloating and gas. People who have little lactase in their bodies can still consume large amounts of milk if it has been allowed to go sour, if lactobacilli have split most of the lactose into lactic acid (as in yogurt), or if the lactose has been treated with commercially available lactase. People originating in northern Europe usually retain full intestinal lactase activity into adult life.

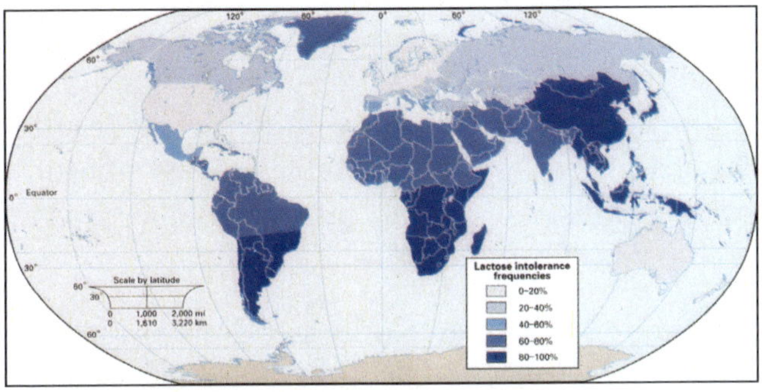

Lactose intolerance, global distribution.

Most commercially available milk has been pasteurized with heat to kill bovine tuberculosis organisms and other possible pathogens. The most widely used method for pasteurizing milk is the high-temperature, short-time (HTST) sterilization treatment. If products are to be stored under refrigeration, or even at room temperature, for long periods of time, they may be processed by ultrahigh temperature (UHT) pasteurization. Another method of preserving milk without refrigeration involves the removal of water to form condensed milk, which can be exposed to air for several days without deterioration. Milk, either whole or defatted, can also be dried to a powder. In some countries, such as the United States, milk is homogenized so that fat particles are broken up and evenly distributed throughout the product.

Cow's milk is good food for human adults, but the cream (i.e., the fat) contains 52 percent saturated fatty acids as compared with only 3 percent polyunsaturated fat. This fat is either drunk with the milk or eaten in butter or cream. Because milk fat is regarded as undesirable by people who want to reduce their energy intake or cholesterol level, the dairy industry has developed low-fat cow's milk (with 2 percent fat instead of the almost 4 percent of whole milk), very low-fat skim milk, and skim milk with extra nonfat milk solids (lactose, protein, and calcium) that give more body to the milk. Buttermilk, originally the watery residue of butter making, is now made from either low-fat or skim milk that has been inoculated with nonpathogenic bacteria.

Cheese making is an ancient art formerly used on farms to convert surplus milk into a food that could be stored without refrigeration. Rennet, an enzyme found in a calf's stomach, is added to milk, causing the milk protein casein to coagulate into a semisolid substance called curd, thus trapping most of the fat. The remaining watery liquid (whey) is then drained, and the curd is salted, inoculated with nonpathogenic organisms, and allowed to dry and mature. Cheese is rich in protein and calcium and is a good source of vitamin A and riboflavin. Most cheeses, however, contain about 25 to 30 percent fat (constituting about 70 percent of the calories of the cheese), which is mostly saturated, and they are usually high in sodium.

Fats and Oils

The animal fats used by humans are butter, suet (beef fat), lard (pork fat), and fish oils. Important vegetable oils include olive oil, peanut (groundnut) oil, coconut oil, cottonseed oil, sunflower seed oil, soybean oil, safflower oil, rape oil, sesame (gingelly) oil, mustard oil, red palm oil, and corn oil. Fats and oils provide more calories per gram than any other food, but they contain no protein and few micronutrients. Vitamins A and D are added to margarines. All natural fats and oils contain variable amounts of vitamin E, the fat-soluble vitamin antioxidant.

The predominant substances in fats and oils are triglycerides, chemical compounds containing any three fatty acids combined with a molecule of glycerol. When no double bonds are present, a fatty acid is said to be saturated; with the presence of one or more double bonds, a fatty acid is said to be unsaturated. Fats with a high percentage of saturated fatty acids, e.g., butter and lard, tend to be solid at room temperature. Those with a high percentage of unsaturated fatty acids are usually liquid oils, e.g., sunflower, safflower, and corn oils. The process of hydrogenation is used by the food industry to convert unsaturated oils to saturated solid fats, which are more resistant to rancidity. However, hydrogenation also causes the formation of trans-fatty acids. These appear to have some of the same undesirable effects on blood cholesterol as saturated fatty acids.

A small group of fatty acids is essential in the diet. They occur in body structures, especially the different membranes inside and around cells, and cannot be synthesized in the body from other fats. Linoleic acid is the most important of these fatty acids because it is convertible to other essential fatty acids. Linoleic acid has two double bonds and is a polyunsaturated fatty acid. As well as being an essential fatty acid, it tends to lower the cholesterol level in the blood. Linoleic acid occurs in moderate to high proportions in many of the seed oils, e.g., corn, sunflower, cottonseed, and safflower oils. Some margarines (polyunsaturated margarines) use a blend of oils selected to provide a moderately high linoleic acid content.

Beverages

Although most adults drink one to two litres (about one to two quarts) of water a day, much of this is in the form of liquids such as coffee, tea, fruit juices, and soft drinks. In general, these are appreciated more for their taste or for their effects than for their nutritive value. Fruit juices are useful for their vitamin C content and are good sources of potassium; however, they tend to be very high in sugar. Coffee and tea by themselves are of little nutritive value; coffee contains some niacin, and tea contains fluoride and manganese. These beverages also contain natural caffeine, which has a stimulating effect. Caffeine is added to colas, and so-called diet soft drinks contain small quantities of artificial sweeteners in place of sugars so that their overall calorie value is reduced.

Since ethyl alcohol (ethanol) has an energy value of 7 kilocalories per gram, very significant amounts of energy can be obtained from alcoholic drinks. Beer contains 2 to 6 percent alcohol, wines 10 to 13 percent, and most spirits up to 40 percent. Fermented drinks also include significant amounts of residual sugars, and champagne and dessert wines may have sugar added to them. With one or two exceptions, alcoholic beverages contain no nutrients and are only a source of "empty calories". The only vitamin present in significant amounts in beer is riboflavin. Wines are devoid of vitamins but sometimes contain large amounts of iron, probably acquired from iron vessels used in their preparation. Heavy alcohol consumption is known to lead to a greater risk of malnutrition, in part because it can damage the absorptive power of the gut and also because heavy drinkers commonly neglect to follow a normal pattern of meals. On the other hand, evidence from a number of studies shows that persons consuming one to two drinks per day are healthier than are those who abstain from drinking alcohol. This might be due in part to substances in red wine, such as flavonoids and tannins, which may protect against heart disease.

Comparison of energy, carbohydrates and alcohol in some common beverages				
Beverage	Typical volume (fl oz)	Energy (kcal)	Carbohydrates (g)	Alcohol (g)
Beer	12	100–150	3–15	12
Club soda	12	0	0	0
Cocktails	3.5	120–180	4–8	18–24
Colas	12	150	40	0
Colas, Diet	12	2	0	0
Ginger Ale	12	120	30	0
Milk, Whole	8	150	11	0

Milk, Skim	8	85	12	0
Spirits	1.5	100–120	0	15–17
Wine, Dessert	3.5	130–160	4–12	11
Wine, Dry	3.5	70–80	3–4	11

Dietary and Nutrient Recommendations

Notions of what constitutes a healthful diet vary with geography and custom as well as with changing times and an evolving understanding of nutrition. In the past, people had to live almost entirely on food that was locally produced. With industrialization and globalization, however, food can now be transported over long distances. Researchers must be careful in making generalizations about a national diet from a relatively small sample of the population; the poor cannot afford to eat the same diet as the rich, and many countries have large immigrant groups with their own distinctive food patterns. Even within a culture, some people abstain on moral or religious grounds from eating certain foods. In general, persons living in more affluent countries eat more meat and other animal products. By comparison, the diets of those living in poorer, agricultural countries rely primarily on cereals in the form of wheat flour, white rice, or corn, with animal products providing less than 10 percent of energy. Another difference between cultures is the extent to which dairy products are consumed. The Chinese, for example, obtain about 2 percent of their energy from dairy products. In contrast, in Pakistan dairy products contribute almost 10 percent of energy. Among Western diets, the lowest in saturated fat is the so-called Mediterranean diet. In the 1950s it was found that Europeans living in rural areas near the Mediterranean Sea had a greater life expectancy than those living elsewhere in Europe, despite poor medical services and a lower standard of living. The traditional diet of Mediterranean peoples is low in animal products; instead, olive oil is a major source of monounsaturated fat. Also, tomatoes and green leafy vegetables, which are regularly consumed in large quantities in the region, contain a variety of antioxidant compounds that are thought to be healthful.

Dietary Guidelines

Following the publication of dietary goals for the Nordic countries in 1968 and for the United States in 1977, dietary goals and guidelines have been set forth by a number of countries and revised periodically as a way of translating scientific recommendations into simple and practical dietary suggestions. These authoritative statements—some published by scientific bodies and some by government agencies—aim to promote long-term health and to prevent or reduce the chances of developing chronic and degenerative diseases. Although the guidelines of different countries may vary in important ways, most recent dietary recommendations include variations on the following fundamental themes: eat a variety of foods; perform regular physical activity and maintain a healthy weight; limit consumption of saturated fat, trans fat, sugar, salt (more specifically, sodium), and alcohol; and emphasize vegetables, fruits, and whole grains.

Food Guide Pyramids and Other Aids

Different formats for dietary goals and guidelines have been developed over the years as educational tools, grouping foods of similar nutrient content together to help facilitate the selection of a balanced diet. In the United States, the four food-group plan of the 1950s—which suggested a milk group, a meat group, a fruit and vegetable group, and a breads and cereals group as a basic diet—was replaced in 1992 by the five major food groups of the Food Guide Pyramid. This innovative visual display was introduced by the United States Department of Agriculture (USDA) as a tool for helping the public cultivate a daily pattern of wise food choices, ranging from liberal consumption of grain products, as represented in the broad base of the pyramid, to sparing use of fats, oils, and sugary foods, as represented in the apex. Subsequently, similar devices were developed for particular cultural and ethnic food patterns such as Asian, Latin American, Mediterranean, and even vegetarian diets—all emphasizing grains, vegetables, and fruits. While an adaptation of the 1992 USDA pyramid was used by Mexico, Chile, the Philippines, and Panama, a rainbow was used by Canada, a square by Zimbabwe, plates by Australia and the United Kingdom, a bean pot by Guatemala, the number 6 by Japan, and a pagoda by South Korea and China.

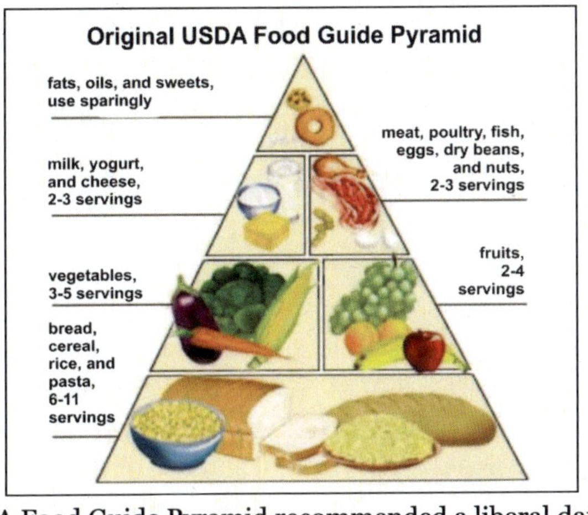

The original USDA Food Guide Pyramid recommended a liberal daily intake of grain products (represented by the wide base of the pyramid) and a sparing intake of fats, oils, and sugary foods (represented by the tip of the structure).

In the early 21st century, many countries altered the pictorial representation of their food guides. For example, in 2005 Japan introduced a spinning-top food guide that essentially was an inverted version of the U.S. pyramid graphic. That same year, the USDA released new dietary guidelines and redesigned its original Food Guide Pyramid, which was known as MyPyramid and featured colourful vertical stripes of varying widths to reflect the relative proportions of different food groups. Similar to Japan's spinning-top graphic, which depicted a figure running on the top's upper level, the MyPyramid graphic used a figure climbing steps to illustrate the importance of daily exercise. Unlike the original Food Guide Pyramid, the abstract geometry of MyPyramid did not offer specific dietary guidance at a glance; rather, individuals were directed to an interactive web site for customized eating plans based on their age, sex, and activity level.

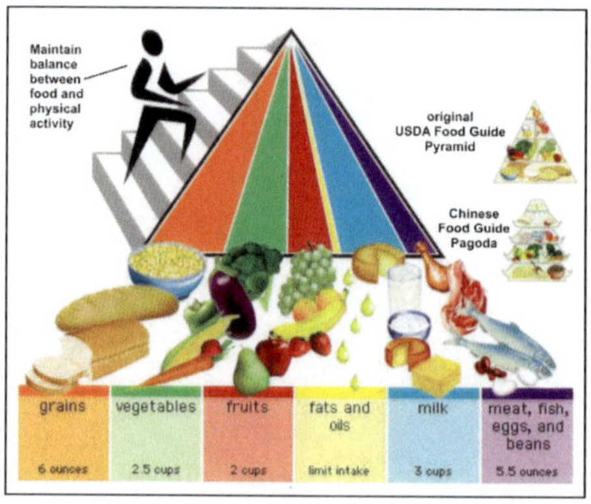

2005 U.S. Food Guide Pyramid.

In 2011 the USDA abandoned MyPyramid and introduced MyPlate, which divided the four basic food groups (fruits, grains, protein, and vegetables) into sections on a plate, with the size of each section representing the relative dietary proportions of each food group. A small circle shown at the edge of the plate was used to illustrate the dietary inclusion and proportion of dairy products. Unlike MyPyramid, MyPlate did not include an exercise component, nor did it include a section for fats and oils. The two were similar, however, in that the guidance they offered was nonspecific and was supported by a web site.

Adapting Guidelines to Culture

Dietary guidelines have been largely the province of more affluent countries, where correcting imbalances due to overconsumption and inappropriate food choices has been key. Not until 1989 were proposals for dietary guidelines published from the perspective of low-income countries, such as India, where the primary nutrition problems stemmed from the lack of opportunity to acquire or consume needed food. But even in such countries, there was a growing risk of obesity and chronic disease among the small but increasing number of affluent people who had adopted some of the dietary habits of the industrialized world. For example, the Chinese Dietary Guidelines, published by the Chinese Nutrition Society in 1997, made recommendations for that part of the population dealing with nutritional diseases such as those resulting from iodine and vitamin A deficiencies, for people in some remote areas where there was a lack of food, as well as for the urban population coping with changing lifestyle, dietary excess, and increasing rates of chronic disease. The Food Guide Pagoda, a graphic display intended to help Chinese consumers put the dietary recommendations into practice, rested on the traditional cereal-based Chinese diet. Those who could not tolerate fresh milk were encouraged to consume yogurt or other dairy products as a source of calcium. Unlike dietary recommendations in Western countries, the pagoda did not include sugar, as sugar consumption by the Chinese was quite low; however, children and adolescents in particular were cautioned to limit sugar intake because of the risk of dental caries.

Nutrient Recommendations

Standards for evaluating the adequacy of specific nutrients in an individual diet or the diet of a population require more detailed and quantitative recommendations. Nutrient recommendations are usually determined by scientific bodies within a country at the behest of government agencies. The World Health Organization and other agencies of the United Nations have also issued reports on nutrients and food components. The Recommended Dietary Allowances (RDAs), first published by the U.S. National Academy of Sciences in 1941 and revised every few years until 1989, established dietary standards for evaluating nutritional intakes of populations and for planning food supplies. The RDAs reflected the best scientific judgment of the time in setting amounts of different nutrients adequate to meet the nutritional needs of most healthy people.

Dietary Reference Intakes

During the 1990s a paradigm shift took place as scientists from the United States and Canada joined forces in an ambitious multiyear project to reframe dietary standards for the two countries. In the revised approach, known as the Dietary Reference Intakes (DRIs), classic indicators of deficiency, such as scurvy and beriberi, were considered an insufficient basis for recommendations. Where warranted by a sufficient research base, the guidelines rely on indicators with broader significance, those that might reflect a decreased risk of chronic diseases such as osteoporosis, heart disease, hypertension, or cancer. DRIs are intended to help individuals plan a healthful diet as well as avoid consuming too much of a nutrient. The comprehensive approach of the DRIs has served as a model for other countries. A DRI report was published in 1997, and subsequent updates were published for specific nutrients and for some food components such as flavonoids that are not considered nutrients but have an impact on health.

The collective term Dietary Reference Intakes encompasses four categories of reference values. The Estimated Average Requirement (EAR) is the intake level for a nutrient at which the needs of 50 percent of the population will be met. Because the needs of the other half of the population will not be met by this amount, the EAR is increased by about 20 percent to arrive at the RDA. The RDA is the average daily dietary intake level sufficient to meet the nutrient requirement of nearly all (97 to 98 percent) healthy persons in a particular life stage. When the EAR, and thus the RDA, cannot be set due to insufficient scientific evidence, another parameter, the Adequate Intake (AI), is given, based on estimates of intake levels of healthy populations. Lastly, the Tolerable Upper Intake Level (UL) is the highest level of a daily nutrient intake that will most likely present no risk of adverse health effects in almost all individuals in the general population.

Tolerable upper intake level (UL) for selected nutrients for adults	
Nutrient	UL per day
Calcium	2,500 milligrams
Copper	10 milligrams
Fluoride	10 milligrams
Folic acid	1,000 micrograms
Iodine	1,100 micrograms
Iron	45 milligrams
Magnesium	350 milligrams
Manganese	11 milligrams
Niacin	35 milligrams
Phosphorus	4 grams
Selenium	400 micrograms
Vitamin A	3,000 micrograms (10,000 IU)
Vitamin B	100 milligrams
Vitamin C	2,000 milligrams
Vitamin D	50 micrograms (2,000 IU)
Vitamin E	1,000 milligrams
Zinc	40 milligrams

Nutrition information is commonly displayed on food labels, but this information is generally simplified to avoid confusion. Because only one nutrient reference value is listed, and because sex and age categories usually are not taken into consideration, the amount chosen is generally the highest RDA value. In the United States, for example, the Daily Values, determined by the Food and Drug Administration, are generally based on RDA values published in 1968. The different food components are listed on the food label as a percentage of their Daily Values.

Confidence that a desirable level of intake is reasonable for a particular group of people can be bolstered by multiple lines of evidence pointing in the same direction, an understanding of the function of the nutrient and how it is handled by the body, and a comprehensive theoretical model with strong statistical underpinnings. Of critical importance in estimating nutrient requirements is explicitly defining the criterion that the specified level of intake is intended to satisfy. Approaches that use different definitions of adequacy are not comparable. For example, it is one thing to prevent clinical impairment of bodily function (basal requirement), which does not necessarily require any reserves of the nutrient, but it is another to consider an amount that will provide desirable reserves (normative requirement) in the body. Yet another approach attempts to evaluate a nutrient intake conducive to optimal health, even if an amount is required beyond that normally obtainable in food—possibly necessitating the use of supplements. Furthermore, determining upper levels of safe intake requires evidence of a different sort. These issues are extremely complex, and the scientists who collaborate to set nutrient recommendations face exceptional challenges in their attempts to reach consensus.

Sports Nutrition

Sports nutrition is a broad interdisciplinary field that involves dietitians, biochemists, exercise physiologists, cell and molecular biologists, and occasionally psychotherapists. It has both a basic science aspect that includes such concerns as understanding the body's use of nutrients during athletic competition and the need for nutritional supplements among athletes; and an application aspect, which is concerned with the use of proper nutrition and dietary supplements to enhance an athlete's performance. The psychological or psychiatric dimension of sports nutrition is concerned with eating and other mental disorders related to nutrition among athletes.

Some persons who specialize in the field of sports nutrition are registered dietitians (RDs) who have pursued a master's or other advanced degree in the field of exercise physiology; the American Dietetic Association (ADA) has a dietetic practice group or DPG for sports nutritionists called Sports, Cardiovascular, and Wellness Nutritionists (SCAN), which has its own website and telephone contact number.

Fluid Intake Guidelines

Recommended fluid intake for athletes.

Time in reference to event	Ounces of fluid (oz.)
24 hours before	Drink freely
2 hours before	8–16 oz.
15 minutes before	8–16 oz.
During	4 to 8 oz. every 15–20 minutes
After	Drink freely

Purpose

Sports nutrition has several purposes:

- To prepare athletes before performance or training.
- To maintain an acceptable level of performance during competition or training.
- To help the athlete's body recover after training or athletic competition.

- To provide sound information about healthy dietary practices and use of supplements.
- To monitor athletes for signs of eating disorders, doping, supplement abuse, or other unhealthful nutritional practices.
- To provide specialized nutritional advice to athletes following vegetarian, vegan, or other special diets.
- To monitor the special nutritional needs of persons with disabilities who participate in athletic activities and programs.

Hydration

Hydration, or maintaining a proper level of fluid in the body, is an important aspect of sports nutrition because of the loss of water and sodium through sweating during athletic activity. Dehydration results in loss of muscle strength, difficulty concentrating, irritability, and headache.

- Amenorrhea: Absence or suppression of normal menstrual periods in women of childbearing age, usually defined as three to six missed periods.
- Bioelectrical impedance analysis (BIA): A technique for evaluating body composition by passing a small amount of electrical current through the body and measuring the resistance of different types of tissue.
- Body dysmorphic disorder: A mental disorder involving extreme preoccupation with some feature of one's appearance. Excessive time spent in physical exercise, often involving bodybuilding or weight-lifting practices, is a common symptom of the disorder in adolescents.
- Creatine: An organic acid formed and stored in the body that supplies energy to muscle cells. Meat and fish are good dietary sources of creatine.
- Doping: The use of performance-enhancing drugs in sports competition, including anabolic steroids and other substances banned by most international sports organizations. The English word is thought to come from the Dutch dop, which was the name of an alcoholic beverage drunk by Zulu warriors before a battle.
- Electrolyte: Any of several chemicals dissolved in blood and other body fluids that are capable of conducting an electric current. The most important electrolytes in humans and other animals are sodium, potassium, calcium, magnesium, chloride, phosphate, and hydrogen carbonate.
- Ergogenic: Enhancing physical performance, particularly during athletic activity.

- Erythropoetin (EPO): A hormone produced by the kidneys that regulates the production of red blood cells. It is sometimes used by athletes to increase the oxygen-carrying capacity of their blood.
- Female athlete triad: A group of three disorders often found together in female athletes, consisting of disordered eating, amenorrhea, and osteoporosis.
- Glycogen: A complex sugar that is the primary form in which glucose is stored in muscle and liver tissue. Purging—A behavior associated with eating disorders that includes self-induced vomiting and abuse of laxatives as well as diuretics.
- Sports drink: Any beverage containing carbohydrates, electrolytes, and other nutrients as well as water, intended to help athletes rehydrate after training or competition. Sports drinks are isotonic, which means that they contain the same proportion of water, electrolytes, and carbohydrates as the human body.
- Vegan: A vegetarian who excludes all animal products from the diet, including those that can be obtained without killing the animal. Vegans are also known as strict vegetarians.
- Water intoxication: A potentially fatal condition that occurs when an athlete loses sodium from the body through perspiration and drinks a large quantity of water in a short period of time without replacing the sodium. Long-distance runners are particularly susceptible to water intoxication.

Initial body weight through sweating without replacing the lost fluid is at risk of heat cramps, heat exhaustion, and heat stroke. Moreover, dehydration may be progressive in athletes who do not replace fluid loss overnight; the greater the loss of body fluid, the longer it takes to rehydrate the body. When dehydration has taken place over 2 to 3 days, it will take a minimum of 48 hours to replace the fluids in body tissues. The health risks of dehydration are a major reason why abuse of diuretics is dangerous in athletes.

People vary in their sweating rates; therefore, health professionals must evaluate athletes on an individual basis to determine how much fluid is needed after exercise or training. The most common way to measure this need is to weigh the athlete before and after exercise; the amount of weight lost should be replaced with an equal amount of fluid before the next workout. The usual rule of thumb is 1 pint of fluid containing carbohydrates and electrolytes for each pound of weight loss.

Good hydration is more effectively maintained by consuming sports drinks or other beverages that contain salt and carbohydrates than by drinking plain water. Sports drinks are isotonic; that is, they contain the same proportion of electrolytes and carbohydrates to fluid as the human body. After exercise, the body requires carbohydrates to replace the glycogen (a complex sugar) stored in muscle tissue and the liver. Glycogen is an important source of reserve energy for muscles; long-distance runners who deplete their stores of glycogen may experience fatigue to the point of being unable to move. In addition to the risk of glycogen depletion, drinking only water places the athlete at risk of water intoxication, a potentially fatal condition in which the sodium lost through sweat is not replaced and is followed by the rapid intake of a large quantity of water. The resulting electrolyte imbalance affects the brain and central nervous system. Blood plasma sodium levels below 100 mmol/L (2.3g/L) frequently result in swelling of the brain tissue, coma, and even death.

Assessment of Energy Needs

Athletes usually require a higher level of calorie intake than nonathletes, although the amount varies depending on the athlete's sex, age, height, weight, body composition, stage of growth, level of fitness, and the intensity, frequency, and duration of physical exercise. An appropriate diet for most athletes consists of a minimum of 2000 calories per day; 55–65% should come from carbohydrates, 15–20% from protein, and 20–30% from fats.

Assessment of Weight and Body Composition

The use of the body mass index (BMI) to evaluate athletes' weight is not recommended because many have a high proportion of muscle tissue to fat and may therefore be considered "overweight" by standard body mass charts. A better reference guide is to check whether the athlete falls between the 25th and the 75th percentile of weight for height by age, measured according to the National Center for Health Statistics (NCHS) guidelines.

Well-nourished athletes should have a lean muscle mass above the 25th percentile, although the ideal ratio of lean muscle to body fat has not yet been established for any sport. Male athletes, however, should not have less than 7% body fat. There are several methods for estimating the proportion of body fat on an athlete's body: underwater weighing (equipment is expensive and limited in availability); skinfold measurements taken by high-precision calipers on three to five sites on the right side of the body (the right side is always used even if the athlete is left-handed); bioelectrical impedance analysis or BIA (a technique that measures body composition by passing a small electrical current through the body and measuring the resistance of various body tissues, as lean muscle contains a higher proportion of water than fat); and computerized calipers.

Strategies for Weight Change

It is important for athletes in any age group needing or desiring to lose or gain weight to be properly supervised by a nutritionist as well as a physician, because unhealthful dietary practices can lead to long-term mental as well as physical disorders. The American Academy of Pediatrics (AAP) makes the following recommendations for weight change in young athletes:

- The dietary program should be started in a timely fashion to permit gradual weight gain or loss over a reasonable time period.
- The program should allow a gain or loss of no more than 1.5% of body weight per week.
- It should be designed to permit weight lost to be fat and weight gained to be muscle.
- It should be accompanied by appropriate strength and conditioning training.
- The diet should provide an appropriate balance of carbohydrates, protein, and fats.

Weight Loss

Weight loss programs are sometimes recommended for athletes in weight-sensitive sports, most often wrestling or judo for boys and figure skating, gymnastics, long-distance running, rowing, and swimming for girls. Unfortunately, many young people go too far in adopting unhealthful eating or exercise patterns in order to keep their weight down. Because of this tendency, the AAP states that children younger than the ninth grade should not be put on weight-loss regimens to improve athletic performance.

Restricting food intake is the most common method of weight loss among athletes, but a large percentage of young athletes also engage in purging (self-induced vomiting plus abuse of laxatives and diuretics), fasting, or the use of stimulants, wet suits, sauna baths, or compulsive exercising. Some studies have shown that as many as 11% of wrestlers meet the criteria for eating disorders, and 15% of swimmers.

Unhealthful weight loss practices are dangerous because much of the weight lost will be lean muscle rather than fat, which can affect athletic performance. Girls who develop eating disorders or body dysmorphic disorder are at risk of developing the so-called female athlete triad, which consists of disordered eating, cessation of menstrual periods (amenorrhea), and osteoporosis or brittle bones. A common symptom associated with the triad is an unusually high number of stress fractures during the girl's athletic career. The triad, which was first described in 1993, may have long-term consequences for a woman's health. Female athletes in their freshman year of college are reported to be at increased risk of developing the triad, particularly if it is their first experience of living away from home or they are having academic difficulties.

Weight Gain

Athletes in sports requiring strength or weight lifting (football, rugby, basketball, bodybuilding) may try to gain weight in order to build the body's muscle mass. Inappropriate methods, however, will lead to gaining fat rather than muscle, putting the athlete at risk in midlife for high blood pressure, cardiovascular disease, and type 2 diabetes. It is important for athletes to recognize the genetic limitations related to their body build, as persons who are naturally slender cannot add as much muscle tissue to their bodies as those who are built more solidly.

The safest way to gain weight and build muscle tissue is to consume 1.5 to 1.75 grams of protein per kilogram of body weight per day and participate in strength training. The most effective form of strength training is thought to be multiple sets of weight lifting with a relatively high number of repetitions (8–15) per set. Athletes should avoid the use of dietary supplements in building muscle, particularly steroids, which have been shown to be harm-fultohealthinboth males and females.

Use of Ergogenic Aids

Ergogenic aids are drugs or dietary supplements taken to improve athletic performance or endurance by providing energy or adding muscle tissue. The most common ergogenic aids used are anabolic or andro-genic steroids (male sex hormones), steroid precursors, growth hormone, creatine (an organic acid stored in the body that supplies energy to muscle cells), and ephedra, an herb sometimes called by its Chinese name, ma huang. Some ergogenic aids are illegal to use in competition.

Medical and nutritional professionals are concerned about the use of ergogenic aids among young athletes for two major reasons. The first is that these drugs and supplements, first used by adult athletes in the 1980s, are now being used by children as young as 10 or 12. The second is that creatine and anabolic steroids may produce long-term adverse effects on the body even though they do produce gains in body mass and strength, while steroid precursors, ephedra, and growth hormone pose a good many risks to health without any proof that they enhance athletic performance.

The ADA's position statement says, "Nutritional ergogenic aids should be used with caution, and only after careful evaluation of the product for safety, efficacy, potency, and whether or not it is a banned or illegal substance".

Precautions

Consultation with a qualified sports nutritionist is a sound practice for anyone in any age group who is heavily involved in any sport, whether amateur or professional. Specific precautions:

- Consultation should be individualized, as people vary in their energy needs, sweating rates, body composition, etc.

- Any female athlete who stops having menstrual periods (amenorrhea) or has only scanty periods (oligomenorrhea) should be evaluated for disordered eating.
- Nutritional advice should be given by a registered dietitian or physician, not by a coach. The American Academy of Pediatrics notes that "most coaches do not have an adequate nutritional background to counsel an athlete about weight loss".
- Coaches should avoid discussing weight loss with young athletes (with the exception of sports requiring weigh-ins before competition), as such discussions often lead to the athlete's use of harmful weight-loss practices.
- Athletes should not take any dietary supplement without consulting their physician and a nutritionist.
- Athletes following a vegetarian or vegan diet require special attention to protein and iron intake.

Interactions

Some herbal dietary supplements used by athletes are known to interact with prescription medications, such as St. John's wort (Hypericum perforatum) and ephedra (Ephedra sinica), often used to promote weight loss; valerian (Valeriana officinalis),often taken for insomnia; cayenne (Capsicum frutescens), ginseng (Panax ginseng), and cordyceps (Cordyceps sinensis), taken internally to increase carbohydrate metabolism or increase endurance; and Siberian ginseng (Eleutherococcus senticosus) and echinacea (Echinacea angustifolia), taken to boost the immune system. Some of these drug interactions are potentially serious. Athletes should not take any herbal remedies, including those marketed specifically to athletes, without consulting their physician and a nutritionist.

Complications

There are no complications associated with nutritional monitoring of athletes by qualified professionals. The AAP, however, recommends seeking nutritional information and assessment from dietetics professionals, not from team coaches or personal trainers.

Parental Concerns

Parental concerns about sports nutrition are age-related in most cases. Parents of young children should be aware of the ways in which children's hydration requirements during athletic activity differ from those of adults. Parents of adolescents who are heavily involved in sports should acquaint themselves with the signs of unhealthy eating or dieting practices in high school or college-age athletes.

Hydration Needs in Young Children

Young children are more susceptible to heat-related illnesses than adults during exercise for several reasons: they produce more heat relative to body mass for the same intensity of exercise; they have a lower cardiac output than adults at any exercise level; they have a higher threshold for rise in body temperature before beginning to sweat; and they have a lower sweating capacity than adults, which makes it harder for them to dissipate body heat through evaporation. Children also have a less efficient thirst mechanism than adults, which means that they are more likely to become dehydrated during exercise because they do not feel as intense a need to drink liquids. Orange- or grape-flavored drinks are often a good way to rehydrate children because they will increase their fluid intake when the beverage is flavored.

Female Athlete Triad

Parents should watch for indications of the female athlete triad, such as missing three or more menstrual periods; an unusual number of stress fractures; an excessive amount of time spent exercising or working out; a tendency to wear baggy or concealing clothes even in warm weather; and a restricted eating pattern. Adopting a vegetarian or vegan diet may indicate the onset of an eating disorder in a female athlete.

Doping

Doping in sports refers to the practice of taking anabolic steroids and other substances forbidden by international sports organizations. The word is derived from the Dutch word for an alcoholic drink consumed by Zulu warriors to give them energy before a battle. In the early twentieth century, doping referred primarily to the illegal drugging of race horses, but has been applied to human athletes since the 1920s.

In the 1970s, testing of athletes' blood samples focused largely on steroid use, but in the 1980s and 1990s, new tests had to be devised to detect evidence of blood doping. Blood doping refers to the use of blood transfusions or a hormone called erythropoetin (EPO) in order to increase the level of hemoglobin in an athlete's blood, and therefore its oxygen-carrying capacity. The use of EPO in such endurance sports as marathon running or cycling increases the athlete's risk of heart disease if it is used to raise blood hemoglobin levels above 13.0 g/dL.

Newer forms of doping include the use of modafinil (Provigil), a drug ordinarily used to treat narcolepsy (a sleep disorder), and gene doping. Gene doping is defined by the World Anti-Doping Agency, an organization founded in 1999, as "the non-therapeutic use of cells, genes, genetic elements, or of the modulation of gene expression, having the capacity to improve athletic performance." One possible technique of gene doping would be the use of a synthetic gene that could last for years and produce high amounts of naturally occurring muscle-building hormones.

Vegetarian and Vegan Diets

It is possible for an athlete to maintain strength and overall health on a vegetarian diet provided that a variety of plant-based sources of protein are consumed on a daily basis and energy intake is adequate. Vegetarian and especially vegan athletes are at risk of inadequate creatine and iron intake, however, as well as insufficient amounts of zinc, vitamin B_{12}, vitamin D, and calcium. Iron deficiency will eventually affect athletic performance, as will low levels of creatine. Coaches and trainers should be aware that sudden adoption of a vegetarian or vegan diet in an athlete who was previously eating meat and fish may indicate the onset of an eating disorder.

References

- Introduction-to-nutrition: healthengine.com.au, Retrieved 25 June, 2019
- Human-nutrition, science: britannica.com, Retrieved 08 April, 2019
- Food-groups, human-nutrition, science: britannica.com, Retrieved 27 July, 2019
- Sports-nutrition, encyclopedias-almanacs-transcripts-and-maps, science: encyclopedia.com, Retrieved 14 March, 2019

2

Metabolism and Metabolic Pathways

The set of chemical reactions which are vital for the sustenance of life is known as metabolism. The different metabolic reactions are organized into metabolic pathways, where a chemical is transformed into another chemical through a series of steps. This chapter has been carefully written to provide an easy understanding of the varied facets of metabolism such as microbial metabolism and ATP in metabolism.

Metabolism

Metabolism is the sum of the chemical reactions that take place within each cell of a living organism and that provide energy for vital processes and for synthesizing new organic material.

Living organisms are unique in that they can extract energy from their environments and use it to carry out activities such as movement, growth and development, and reproduction. But how do living organisms—or, their cells—extract energy from their environments, and how do cells use this energy to synthesize and assemble the components from which the cells are made?

The answers to these questions lie in the enzyme-mediated chemical reactions that take place in living matter (metabolism). Hundreds of coordinated, multistep reactions, fueled by energy obtained from nutrients and/or solar energy, ultimately convert readily available materials into the molecules required for growth and maintenance.

The Unity of Life

At the cellular level of organization, the main chemical processes of all living matter are similar, if not identical. This is true for animals, plants, fungi, or bacteria; where variations occur (such as, for example, in the secretion of antibodies by some molds), the variant processes are but variations on common themes. Thus, all living matter is made up of large molecules called proteins, which provide support and coordinated movement, as well as storage and transport of small molecules, and, as catalysts, enable chemical reactions to take place rapidly and specifically under mild temperature, relatively low concentration, and neutral conditions (i.e., neither acidic nor basic). Proteins are assembled from some 20 amino acids, and, just as the 26 letters of the alphabet can be assembled in specific ways to form words of various lengths and meanings, so may tens or even hundreds of the 20 amino-acid "letters" be joined to form specific proteins. Moreover, those portions of protein molecules involved in performing similar functions in different organisms often comprise the same sequences of amino acids.

There is the same unity among cells of all types in the manner in which living organisms preserve their individuality and transmit it to their offspring. For example, hereditary information is encoded in a specific sequence of bases that make up the DNA (deoxyribonucleic acid) molecule in the nucleus of each cell. Only four bases are used in synthesizing DNA: adenine, guanine, cytosine, and thymine. Just as the Morse Code consists of three simple signals—a dash, a dot, and a space—the precise arrangement of which suffices to convey coded messages, so the precise arrangement of the bases in DNA contains and conveys the information for the synthesis and assembly of cell components. Some primitive life-forms, however, use RNA (ribonucleic acid; a nucleic acid differing from DNA in containing the sugar ribose instead of the sugar deoxyribose and the base uracil instead of the base thymine) in place of DNA as a primary carrier of genetic information. The replication of the genetic material in these organisms must, however, pass through a DNA phase. With minor exceptions, the genetic code used by all living organisms is the same.

The chemical reactions that take place in living cells are similar as well. Green plants use the energy of sunlight to convert water (H_2O) and carbon dioxide (CO_2) to carbohydrates (sugars and starches), other organic (carbon-containing) compounds, and molecular oxygen (O_2). The process of photosynthesis requires energy, in the form of sunlight, to split one water molecule into one-half of an oxygen molecule (O_2; the oxidizing agent) and two hydrogen atoms (H; the reducing agent), each of which dissociates to one hydrogen ion (H^+) and one electron. Through a series of oxidation-reduction reactions, electrons (denoted e^-) are transferred from a donating molecule (oxidation), in this case water, to an accepting molecule (reduction) by a series of chemical reactions; this "reducing power" may be coupled ultimately to the reduction of carbon dioxide to the level of carbohydrate. In effect, carbon dioxide accepts and bonds with hydrogen, forming carbohydrates ($C_n[H_2O]_n$).

Living organisms that require oxygen reverse this process: they consume carbohydrates and other organic materials, using oxygen synthesized by plants to form water, carbon dioxide, and energy. The process that removes hydrogen atoms (containing electrons) from the carbohydrates and passes them to the oxygen is an energy-yielding series of reactions.

In plants, all but two of the steps in the process that converts carbon dioxide to carbohydrates are the same as those steps that synthesize sugars from simpler starting materials in animals, fungi, and bacteria. Similarly, the series of reactions that take a given starting material and synthesize certain molecules that will be used in other synthetic pathways are similar, or identical, among all cell types. From a metabolic point of view, the cellular processes that take place in a lion are only marginally different from those that take place in a dandelion.

Biological Energy Exchanges

The energy changes associated with physicochemical processes are the province of thermodynamics, a subdiscipline of physics. The first two laws of thermodynamics state, in essence, that energy can be neither created nor destroyed and that the effect of physical and chemical changes is to increase the disorder, or randomness (i.e., entropy), of the universe. Although it might be supposed that biological processes—through which organisms grow in a highly ordered and complex manner, maintain order and complexity throughout their life, and pass on the instructions for order to succeeding generations—are in contravention of these laws, this is not so. Living organisms neither consume nor create energy: they can only transform it from one form to another. From the environment they absorb energy in a form useful to them; to the environment they return an equivalent amount of energy in a biologically less useful form. The useful energy, or free energy, may be defined as energy capable of doing work under isothermal conditions (conditions in which no temperature differential exists); free energy is associated with any chemical change. Energy less useful than free energy is returned to the environment, usually as heat. Heat cannot perform work in biological systems because all parts of cells have essentially the same temperature and pressure.

The Carrier of Chemical Energy

At any given time, a neutral molecule of water dissociates into a hydrogen ion (H^+) and a hydroxide ion (OH^-), and the ions are continually re-forming into the neutral molecule. Under normal conditions (neutrality), the concentration of hydrogen ions (acidic ions) is equal to that of the hydroxide ions (basic ions); each are at a concentration of 10^{-7} mole per litre, which is described as a pH of 7.

All cells either are bounded by membranes or contain organelles that have membranes. These membranes do not permit water or the ions derived from water to pass into or out of the cells or organelles. In green plants, sunlight is absorbed by chlorophyll and other pigments in the chloroplasts of the cells, called photosystem II. When a water molecule is split by light energy, one-half of an oxygen molecule and two hydrogen atoms (which dissociate to two electrons and two hydrogen ions, H^+) are formed. When excited by sunlight, chlorophyll loses one electron to an electron carrier molecule but quickly recovers it from a hydrogen atom of the split water molecule, which sends H+ into solution in the process. Two oxygen atoms come together to form a molecule of oxygen gas (O_2). The free electrons are passed to photosystem I, but, in doing so, an excess concentration of positively charged hydrogen ions (H^+) appears on one side of the membrane in the chloroplast, whereas an excess of negatively charged hydroxide ions (OH^-) builds up on the other side. The free energy released as H^+ ions move through a specific "pore" in the membrane, to equalize the concentrations of ions, is sufficient to make some biological processes work, such as the uptake of certain nutrients by bacteria and the rotation of the whiplike protein-based propellers that enable such bacteria to move. Equally important, however, is that this gradient across the membrane powers the formation of adenosine triphosphate (ATP) from inorganic phosphate (HPO_4^{2-}, abbreviated Pi) and adenosine diphosphate (ADP). ATP is the major carrier of biologically utilizable energy in all forms of living matter. The interrelationships of energy-yielding and energy-requiring metabolic reactions may be considered largely as processes that couple the formation of ATP with its breakdown.

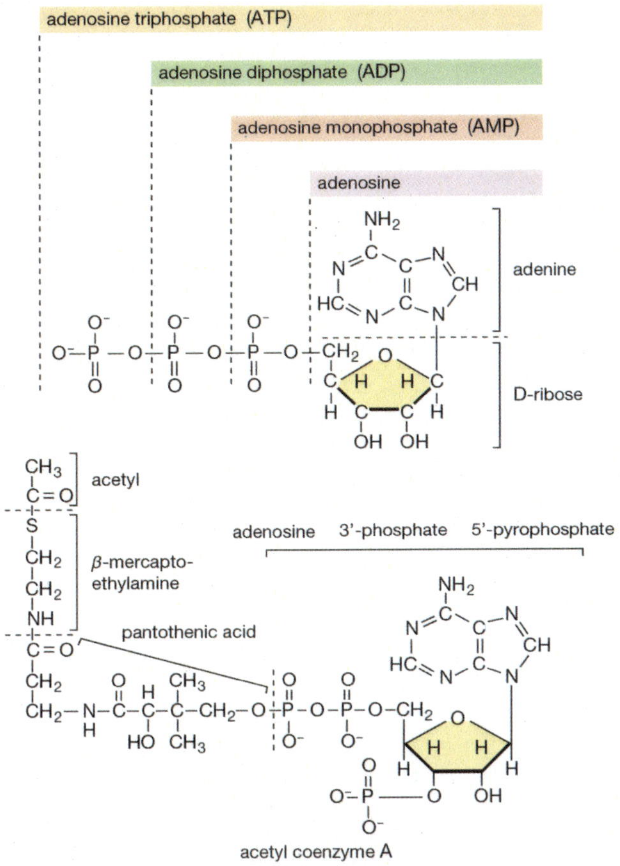

Biological Energy Carriers.

Synthesis of ATP by green plants is similar to the synthesis of ATP that takes place in the mitochondria of animal, plant, and fungus cells, and in the plasma membranes of bacteria that use oxygen (or other inorganic electron acceptors, such as nitrate) to accept electrons from the removal of hydrogen atoms from a molecule of food. Through these processes most of the energy stored in food materials is released and converted into the molecules that fuel life processes. It must also be remembered, however, that many living organisms (usually bacteria and protozoa) cannot tolerate oxygen; they form ATP from inorganic phosphate and ADP by substrate-level phosphorylations (the addition of a phosphate group) that do not involve the establishment and collapse of proton gradients across membranes. It must also be borne in mind that the fuels of life and the cellular "furnace" in which they are "burned" are made of the same types of material: if the fires burn too brightly, not only the fuel but also the furnace is consumed. It is therefore essential to release energy at small, discrete, readily utilizable intervals. The relative complexity of the catabolic pathways (by which food materials are broken down) and the complexity of the anabolic pathways (by which cell components are synthesized) reflect this need and offer the possibility for simple feedback systems to control the rate at which materials travel along these sequences of enzymic reactions.

Catabolism

The release of chemical energy from food materials essentially occurs in three phases. In the first phase (phase I), the large molecules that make up the bulk of food materials are broken down into small constituent units: proteins are converted to the 20 or so different amino acids of which they are composed; carbohydrates (polysaccharides such as starch in plants and glycogen in animals) are degraded to sugars such as glucose; and fats (lipids) are broken down into fatty acids and glycerol. The amounts of energy liberated in phase I are relatively small: only about 0.6 percent of the free, or useful, energy of proteins and carbohydrates, and about 0.1 percent of that of fats, is released during this phase. Because this energy is liberated largely as heat, it cannot be used by the cell. The purpose of the reactions of phase I, which can be grouped under the term digestion and which, in animals, occur mainly in the intestinal tract and in tissues in which reserve materials are prepared, or mobilized, for energy production, is to prepare the foodstuffs for the energy-releasing processes.

Incomplete Oxidation

In the second phase of the release of energy from food (phase II), the small molecules produced in the first phase—sugars, glycerol, a number of fatty acids, and about 20 varieties of amino acids—are incompletely oxidized (in this sense, oxidation means the removal of electrons or hydrogen atoms), the end product being (apart from carbon dioxide and water) one of only three possible substances: the two-carbon compound acetate, in the form of a compound called acetyl coenzyme A; the four-carbon compound oxaloacetate; and the five-carbon compound α-oxoglutarate. The first, acetate in the form of acetyl coenzyme A, constitutes by far the most common product—it is the product of two-thirds of the carbon incorporated into carbohydrates and glycerol; all of the carbon in most fatty acids; and approximately half of the carbon in amino acids. The end product of several amino acids is α-oxoglutarate; that of a few others is oxaloacetate, which is formed either directly or indirectly (from fumarate). These processes occur in animals, plants, bacteria, fungi, and other organisms capable of oxidizing their food materials wholly to carbon dioxide and water.

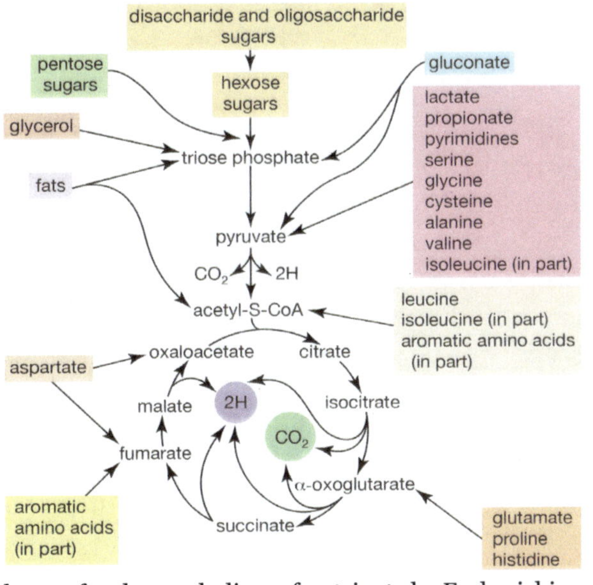

Pathways for the catabolism of nutrients by Escherichia coli.

Complete Oxidation

Total oxidation of the relatively few products of phase II occurs in a cyclic sequence of chemical reactions known as the tricarboxylic acid (TCA) cycle, or the Krebs cycle, after its discoverer, Sir Hans Krebs; it represents phase III of energy release from foods. Each turn of this cycle is initiated by the formation of citrate, with six carbon atoms, from oxaloacetate (with four carbons) and acetyl coenzyme A; subsequent reactions result in the reformation of oxaloacetate and the formation of two molecules of carbon dioxide. The carbon atoms that go into the formation of carbon dioxide are no longer available to the cell. The concomitant stepwise oxidations—in which hydrogen atoms or electrons are removed from intermediate compounds formed during the cycle and, via a system of carriers, are transferred ultimately to oxygen to form water—are quantitatively the most important means of generating ATP from ADP and inorganic phosphate. These events are known as terminal respiration and oxidative phosphorylation.

Some microorganisms, incapable of completely converting their carbon compounds to carbon dioxide, release energy by fermentation reactions, in which the intermediate compounds of catabolic routes either directly or indirectly accept or donate hydrogen atoms. Such secondary changes in intermediate compounds result in considerably less energy being made available to the cell than occurs with the pathways that are linked to oxidative phosphorylation; however, fermentation reactions yield a large variety of commercially important products. Thus, for example, if the oxidation (removal of electrons or hydrogen atoms) of some catabolic intermediate is coupled to the reduction of pyruvate or of acetaldehyde derived from pyruvate, the products formed are lactic acid and ethyl alcohol, respectively.

Anabolism

Catabolic pathways effect the transformation of food materials into interconvertible intermediates. Anabolic pathways, on the other hand, are sequences of enzyme-catalyzed reactions in which the component building blocks of large molecules, or macromolecules (e.g., proteins, carbohydrates, and fats), are constructed from the same intermediates. Thus, catabolic routes have clearly defined beginnings but no unambiguously identifiable end products; anabolic routes, on the other hand, lead to clearly distinguishable end products from diffuse beginnings. The two types of pathway are linked through reactions of phosphate transfer, involving ADP, AMP, and ATP, and also through electron transfers, which enable reducing equivalents (i.e., hydrogen atoms or electrons), which have been released during catabolic reactions, to be utilized for biosynthesis. But, although catabolic and anabolic pathways are closely linked, and although the overall effect of one type of route is obviously the opposite of the other, they have few steps in common. The anabolic pathway for the synthesis of a particular molecule generally starts from intermediate compounds quite different from those produced as a result of catabolism of that molecule; for example, microorganisms catabolize aromatic (i.e., containing a ring, or cyclic, structure) amino acids to acetyl coenzyme A and an intermediate compound of the TCA cycle. The biosynthesis of these amino acids, however, starts with a compound derived from pyruvate and an intermediate compound of the metabolism of pentose (a general name for sugars with five carbon atoms). Similarly, histidine is synthesized from a pentose sugar but is catabolized to α-oxoglutarate.

Even in cases in which a product of catabolism is used in an anabolic pathway, differences emerge; thus, fatty acids, which are catabolized to acetyl coenzyme A, are synthesized not from acetyl coenzyme A directly but from a derivative of it, malonyl coenzyme A. Furthermore, even enzymes that catalyze apparently identical steps in catabolic and anabolic routes may exhibit different properties. In general, therefore, the way down (catabolism) is different from the way up (anabolism). These differences are important because they allow for the regulation of catabolic and anabolic processes in the cell.

In eukaryotic cells (i.e., those with a well-defined nucleus, characteristic of organisms higher than bacteria) the enzymes of catabolic and anabolic pathways are often located in different cellular compartments. This also contributes to the manner of their cellular control; for example, the formation of acetyl coenzyme A from fatty acids, referred to above, occurs in animal cells in small sausage-shaped components, or organelles, called mitochondria, which also contain the enzymes for terminal respiration and for oxidative phosphorylation. The biosynthesis of fatty acids from acetyl coenzyme A, on the other hand, occurs in the cytoplasm.

Integration of Catabolism and Anabolism

Fine Control

Possibly the most important means for controlling the flux of metabolites through catabolic and anabolic pathways, and for integrating the numerous different pathways in the cell, is through the regulation of either the activity or the synthesis of key (pacemaker) enzymes. It was recognized in the 1950s, largely from work with microorganisms, that pacemaker enzymes can interact with small molecules at more than one site on the surface of the enzyme molecule. The reaction between an enzyme and its substrate—defined as the compound with which the enzyme acts to form a product—occurs at a specific site on the enzyme known as the catalytic, or active, site; the proper fit between the substrate and the active site is an essential prerequisite for the occurrence of a reaction catalyzed by an enzyme. Interactions at other, so-called regulatory sites on the enzyme, however, do not result in a chemical reaction but cause changes in the shape of the protein; the changes profoundly affect the catalytic properties of the enzyme, either inhibiting or stimulating the rate of the reaction. Modulation of the activity of pacemaker enzymes may be effected by metabolites of the pathway in which the enzyme acts or by those of another pathway; the process may be described as a "fine control" of metabolism. Very small changes in the chemical environment thus produce important and immediate effects on the rates at which individual metabolic processes occur.

Most catabolic pathways are regulated by the relative proportions of ATP, ADP, and AMP in the cell. It is reasonable to suppose that a pathway that serves to make ATP available for energy-requiring reactions would be less active if sufficient ATP were already present, than if ADP or AMP were to accumulate. The relative amounts of the adenine nucleotides (i.e., ATP, ADP, and AMP) thus modulate the overall rate of catabolic pathways. They do so by reacting with specific regulatory sites on pacemaker enzymes necessary for the catabolic pathways, which do not participate in the anabolic routes that effect the opposite reactions. Similarly, it is reasonable to suppose that many anabolic processes, which require energy, are inhibited by ADP or AMP; elevated levels of these nucleotides may be regarded therefore as cellular distress signals indicating a lack of energy.

Since one way in which anabolic pathways differ from catabolic routes is that the former result in identifiable end products, it is not unexpected that the pacemaker enzymes of many anabolic pathways—particularly those effecting the biosynthesis of amino acids and nucleotides —are regulated by the end products of these pathways or, in cases in which branching of pathways occurs, by end products of each branch. Such pacemaker enzymes usually act at the first step unique to a particular anabolic route. If branching occurs, the first step of each branch is controlled. By this so-called negative feedback system, the cellular concentrations of products determine the rates of their formation, thus ensuring that the cell synthesizes only as much of the products as it needs.

Coarse Control

A second and less immediately responsive, or "coarse," control is exerted over the synthesis of pacemaker enzymes. The rate of protein synthesis reflects the activity of appropriate genes, which contain the information that directs all cellular processes. Coarse control is therefore exerted on genetic material rather than on enzymes. Preferential synthesis of a pacemaker enzyme is particularly required to accommodate a cell to major changes in its chemical milieu. Such changes occur in multicellular organisms only to a minor extent, so that this type of control mechanism is less important in animals than in microorganisms. In the latter, however, it may determine the ease with which a cell previously growing in one nutrient medium can grow after transfer to another. In cases in which several types of organism compete in the same medium for available carbon sources, the operation of coarse controls may well be decisive in ensuring survival.

Alterations in the differential rates of synthesis of pacemaker enzymes in microorganisms responding to changes in the composition of their growth medium also manifest the properties of negative feedback systems. Depending on the nature of the metabolic pathway of which a pacemaker enzyme is a constituent, the manner in which the alterations are elicited may be distinguished. Thus, an increase in the rates at which enzymes of catabolic routes are synthesized results from the addition of inducers—usually compounds that exhibit some structural similarity to the substrates on which the enzymes act. A classic example of an inducible enzyme of this type is β-galactosidase. Escherichia coli growing in nutrient medium containing glucose do not utilize the milk sugar, lactose (glucose-4-β-D-galactoside); however, if the bacteria are placed in a growth medium containing lactose as the sole source of carbon, they synthesize β-galactosidase and can therefore utilize lactose. The reaction catalyzed by the enzyme is the hydrolysis (i.e., breakdown involving water) of lactose to its two constituent sugars, glucose and galactose; the preferential synthesis of the enzyme thus allows the bacteria to use the lactose for growth and energy. Another characteristic of the process of enzyme induction is that it continues only as long as the inducer (in this case, lactose) is present; if cells synthesizing β-galactosidase are transferred to a medium containing no lactose, synthesis of β-galactosidase ceases, and the amount of the enzyme in the cells is diluted as they divide, until the original low level of the enzyme is reestablished.

In contrast, the differential rates of synthesis of pacemaker enzymes of anabolic routes are usually not increased by the presence of inducers. Instead, the absence of small molecules that act to repress enzyme synthesis accelerates enzyme formation. Similar to the fine control processes described above is the regulation by coarse control of many pacemaker enzymes of amino-acid biosynthesis. Like the end product inhibitors, the repressors in these cases also appear to be the amino-acid end products themselves. It is useful to regard the acceleration of the enzyme-forming machinery as the consequence, metaphorically, of either placing a foot on the accelerator or removing it from the brake.

Microbial Metabolism

Microbial metabolism is the means by which a microbe obtains the energy and nutrients (e.g. carbon) it needs to live and reproduce. Microbes use many different types of metabolic strategies and species can often be differentiated from each other based on metabolic characteristics. The specific metabolic properties of a microbe are the major factors in determining that microbe's ecological niche, and often allow for that microbe to be useful in industrial processes or responsible for biogeochemical cycles.

Types

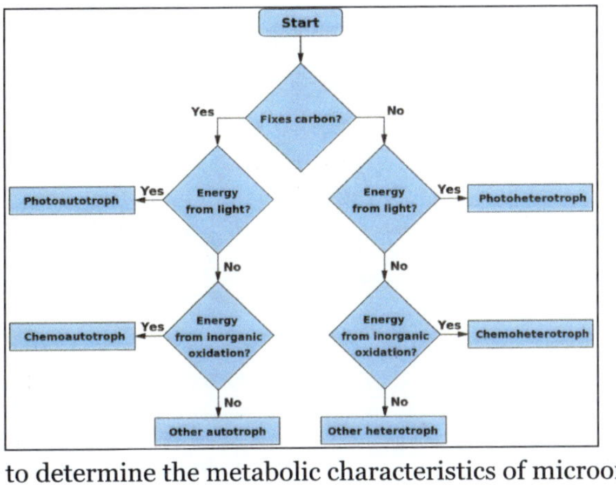

Flow chart to determine the metabolic characteristics of microorganisms.

All microbial metabolisms can be arranged according to three principles:

1. How the organism obtains carbon for synthesising cell mass:

- Autotrophic: Carbon is obtained from carbon dioxide (CO_2).
- Heterotrophic: Carbon is obtained from organic compounds.
- Mixotrophic: Carbon is obtained from both organic compounds and by fixing carbon dioxide.

2. How the organism obtains reducing equivalents used either in energy conservation or in biosynthetic reactions:

- Lithotrophic: Reducing equivalents are obtained from inorganic compounds.
- Organotrophic: Reducing equivalents are obtained from organic compounds.

3. How the organism obtains energy for living and growing:

- Chemotrophic: Energy is obtained from external chemical compounds.
- Phototrophic: Energy is obtained from light.

In practice, these terms are almost freely combined. Typical examples are as follows:

- Chemolithoautotrophs obtain energy from the oxidation of inorganic compounds and carbon from the fixation of carbon dioxide. Examples: Nitrifying bacteria, Sulfur-oxidizing bacteria, Iron-oxidizing bacteria, Knallgas-bacteria.
- Photolithoautotrophs obtain energy from light and carbon from the fixation of carbon dioxide, using reducing equivalents from inorganic compounds. Examples: Cyanobacteria (water (H_2O) as reducing equivalent donor), Chlorobiaceae, Chromatiaceae (hydrogen sulfide (H_2S) as reducing equivalent donor), *Chloroflexus* (hydrogen (H_2) as reducing equivalent donor).
- Chemolithoheterotrophs obtain energy from the oxidation of inorganic compounds, but cannot fix carbon dioxide (CO_2). Examples: some *Thiobacilus*, some *Beggiatoa*, some *Nitrobacter* spp., *Wolinella* (with H_2 as reducing equivalent donor), some Knallgas-bacteria, some sulfate-reducing bacteria.
- Chemoorganoheterotrophs obtain energy, carbon, and reducing equivalents for biosynthetic reactions from organic compounds. Examples: most bacteria, e. g. *Escherichia coli, Bacillus* spp., *Actinobacteria.*
- Photoorganoheterotrophs obtain energy from light, carbon and reducing equivalents for biosynthetic reactions from organic compounds. Some species are strictly heterotrophic, many others can also fix carbon dioxide and are mixotrophic. Examples: *Rhodobacter*, *Rhodopseudomonas*, *Rhodospirillum*, *Rhodomicrobium*, *Rhodocyclus*, *Heliobacterium*, *Chloroflexus* (alternatively to photolithoautotrophy with hydrogen).

Heterotrophic Microbial Metabolism

Some microbes are heterotrophic (more precisely chemoorganoheterotrophic), using organic compounds as both carbon and energy sources. Heterotrophic microbes live off of nutrients that they scavenge from living hosts (as commensals or parasites) or find in dead organic matter of all kind (saprophages). Microbial metabolism is the main contribution for the bodily decay of all organisms after death. Many eukaryotic microorganisms are heterotrophic by predation or parasitism, properties also found in some bacteria such as *Bdellovibrio* (an intracellular parasite of other bacteria, causing death of its victims) and Myxobacteria such as *Myxococcus* (predators of other bacteria which are killed and lysed by cooperating swarms of many single cells of Myxobacteria). Most pathogenic bacteria can be viewed as heterotrophic parasites of humans or the other eukaryotic species they affect. Heterotrophic microbes are extremely abundant in nature and are responsible for the breakdown of large organic polymers such as cellulose, chitin or lignin which are generally indigestible to larger animals. Generally, the breakdown of large polymers to carbon dioxide (mineralization) requires several different organisms, with one breaking down the polymer into its constituent monomers, one able to use the monomers and excreting simpler waste compounds as by-products, and one able to use the excreted wastes. There are many variations on this theme, as different organisms are able to degrade different polymers and secrete different waste products. Some organisms are even able to degrade more recalcitrant compounds such as petroleum compounds or pesticides, making them useful in bioremediation.

Biochemically, prokaryotic heterotrophic metabolism is much more versatile than that of eukaryotic organisms, although many prokaryotes share the most basic metabolic models with eukaryotes, e. g. using glycolysis (also called EMP pathway) for sugar metabolism and the citric acid cycle to degrade acetate, producing energy in the form of ATP and reducing power in the form of NADH or quinols. These basic pathways are well conserved because they are also involved in biosynthesis of many conserved building blocks needed for cell growth (sometimes in reverse direction). However, many bacteria and archaea utilize alternative metabolic pathways other than glycolysis and the citric acid cycle. A well-studied example is sugar metabolism via the keto-deoxy-phosphogluconate pathway (also called ED pathway) in *Pseudomonas*. Moreover, there is a third alternative sugar-catabolic pathway used by some bacteria, the pentose phosphate pathway. The metabolic diversity and ability of prokaryotes to use a large variety of organic compounds arises from the much deeper evolutionary history and diversity of prokaryotes, as compared to eukaryotes. It is also noteworthy that the mitochondrion, the small membrane-bound intracellular organelle that is the site of eukaryotic energy metabolism, arose from the endosymbiosis of a bacterium related to obligate intracellular *Rickettsia*, and also to plant-associated *Rhizobium* or *Agrobacterium*. Therefore, it is not surprising that all mitrochondriate eukaryotes share metabolic properties with these Proteobacteria. Most microbes respire (use an electron transport chain), although oxygen is not the only terminal electron acceptor that may be used. As discussed below, the use of terminal electron acceptors other than oxygen has important biogeochemical consequences.

Special Metabolic Properties

Methylotrophy

Methylotrophy refers to the ability of an organism to use C1-compounds as energy sources. These compounds include methanol, methyl amines, formaldehyde, and formate. Several other less common substrates may also be used for metabolism, all of which lack carbon-carbon bonds. Examples of methylotrophs include the bacteria *Methylomonas* and *Methylobacter*. Methanotrophs are a specific type of methylotroph that are also able to use methane (CH_4) as a carbon source by oxidizing it sequentially to methanol (CH_3OH), formaldehyde (CH_2O), formate ($HCOO^-$), and carbon dioxide CO_2 initially using the enzyme methane monooxygenase. As oxygen is required for this process, all (conventional) methanotrophs are obligate aerobes. Reducing power in the form of quinones and NADH is produced during these oxidations to produce a proton motive force and therefore ATP generation. Methylotrophs and methanotrophs are not considered as autotrophic, because they are able to incorporate some of the oxidized methane (or other metabolites) into cellular carbon before it is completely oxidized to CO_2 (at the level of formaldehyde), using either the serine pathway (*Methylosinus*, *Methylocystis*) or the ribulose monophosphate pathway (*Methylococcus*), depending on the species of methylotroph.

In addition to aerobic methylotrophy, methane can also be oxidized anaerobically. This occurs by a consortium of sulfate-reducing bacteria and relatives of methanogenic Archaea working syntrophically. Little is currently known about the biochemistry and ecology of this process.

Methanogenesis is the biological production of methane. It is carried out by methanogens, strictly anaerobic Archaea such as *Methanococcus*, *Methanocaldococcus*, *Methanobacterium*, *Methanothermus*, *Methanosarcina*, *Methanosaeta* and *Methanopyrus*. The biochemistry of methanogenesis is unique in nature in its use of a number of unusual cofactors to sequentially reduce methanogenic substrates to methane, such as coenzyme M and methanofuran. These cofactors are responsible (among other things) for the establishment of a proton gradient across the outer membrane thereby driving ATP synthesis. Several types of methanogenesis occur, differing in the starting compounds oxidized. Some methanogens reduce carbon dioxide (CO_2) to methane (CH_4) using electrons (most often) from hydrogen gas (H_2) chemolithoautotrophically. These methanogens can often be found in environments containing fermentative organisms. The tight association of methanogens and fermentative bacteria can be considered to be syntrophic because the methanogens, which rely on the fermentors for hydrogen, relieve feedback inhibition of the fermentors by the build-up of excess hydrogen that would otherwise inhibit their growth. This type of syntrophic relationship is specifically known as interspecies hydrogen transfer. A second group of methanogens use methanol (CH_3OH) as a substrate for methanogenesis. These are chemoorganotrophic, but still autotrophic in using CO_2 as only carbon source. The biochemistry of this process is quite different from that of the carbon dioxide-reducing methanogens. Lastly, a third group of methanogens produce both methane and carbon dioxide from acetate (CH_3COO^-) with the acetate being split between the two carbons. These acetate-cleaving organisms are the only chemoorganoheterotrophic methanogens. All autotrophic methanogens use a variation of the reductive acetyl-CoA pathway to fix CO_2 and obtain cellular carbon.

Syntrophy

Syntrophy, in the context of microbial metabolism, refers to the pairing of multiple species to achieve a chemical reaction that, on its own, would be energetically unfavorable. The best studied example of this process is the oxidation of fermentative end products (such as acetate, ethanol and butyrate) by organisms such as *Syntrophomonas*. Alone, the oxidation of butyrate to acetate and hydrogen gas is energetically unfavorable. However, when a hydrogenotrophic (hydrogen-using) methanogen is present the use of the hydrogen gas will significantly lower the concentration of hydrogen (down to 10^{-5} atm) and thereby shift the equilibrium of the butyrate oxidation reaction under standard conditions ($\Delta G^{o\prime}$) to non-standard conditions ($\Delta G'$). Because the concentration of one product is lowered, the reaction is "pulled" towards the products and shifted towards net energetically favorable conditions (for butyrate oxidation: $\Delta G^{o\prime}$= +48.2 kJ/mol, but $\Delta G'$ = -8.9 kJ/mol at 10^{-5} atm hydrogen and even lower if also the initially produced acetate is further metabolized by methanogens). Conversely, the available free energy from methanogenesis is lowered from $\Delta G^{o\prime}$= -131 kJ/mol under standard conditions to $\Delta G'$ = -17 kJ/mol at 10^{-5} atm hydrogen. This is an example of intraspecies hydrogen transfer. In this way, low energy-yielding carbon sources can be used by a consortium of organisms to achieve further degradation and eventual mineralization of these compounds. These reactions help prevent the excess sequestration of carbon over geologic time scales, releasing it back to the biosphere in usable forms such as methane and CO_2.

Anaerobic Respiration

While aerobic organisms during respiration use oxygen as a terminal electron acceptor, anaerobic organisms use other electron acceptors. These inorganic compounds have a lower reduction potential than oxygen, meaning that respiration is less efficient in these organisms and leads to slower growth rates than aerobes. Many facultative anaerobes can use either oxygen or alternative terminal electron acceptors for respiration depending on the environmental conditions.

Most respiring anaerobes are heterotrophs, although some do live autotrophically. All of the processes described below are dissimilative, meaning that they are used during energy production and not to provide nutrients for the cell (assimilative). Assimilative pathways for many forms of anaerobic respiration are also known.

Denitrification – Nitrate as Electron Acceptor

Denitrification is the utilization of nitrate (NO_3^-) as a terminal electron acceptor. It is a widespread process that is used by many members of the Proteobacteria. Many facultative anaerobes use denitrification because nitrate, like oxygen, has a high reduction potential. Many denitrifying bacteria can also use ferric iron (Fe^{3+}) and some organic electron acceptors. Denitrification involves the stepwise reduction of nitrate to nitrite (NO_2^-), nitric oxide (NO), nitrous oxide (N_2O), and dinitrogen (N_2) by the enzymes nitrate reductase, nitrite reductase, nitric oxide reductase, and nitrous oxide reductase, respectively. Protons are transported across the membrane by the initial NADH reductase, quinones, and nitrous oxide reductase to produce the electrochemical gradient critical for respiration. Some organisms (e.g. *E. coli*) only produce nitrate reductase and therefore can accomplish only the first reduction leading to the accumulation of nitrite. Others (e.g. *Paracoccus denitrificans* or *Pseudomonas stutzeri*) reduce nitrate completely. Complete denitrification is an environmentally significant process because some intermediates of denitrification (nitric oxide and nitrous oxide) are important greenhouse gases that react with sunlight and ozone to produce nitric acid, a component of acid rain. Denitrification is also important in biological wastewater treatment where it is used to reduce the amount of nitrogen released into the environment thereby reducing eutrophication. Denitrification can be determined via a nitrate reductase test.

Sulfate Reduction – Sulfate as Electron Acceptor

Dissimilatory sulfate reduction is a relatively energetically poor process used by many Gram-negative bacteria found within the deltaproteobacteria, Gram-positive organisms relating to *Desulfotomaculum* or the archaeon *Archaeoglobus*. Hydrogen sulfide (H_2S) is produced as a metabolic end product. For sulfate reduction electron donors and energy are needed.

Electron Donors

Many sulfate reducers are organotrophic, using carbon compounds such as lactate and pyruvate (among many others) as electron donors, while others are lithotrophic, using hydrogen gas (H_2) as an electron donor. Some unusual autotrophic sulfate-reducing bacteria (e.g. *Desulfotignum phosphitoxidans*) can use phosphite (HPO_3^-) as an electron donor whereas others (e.g. *Desulfovibrio sulfodismutans, Desulfocapsa thiozymogenes, Desulfocapsa sulfoexigens*) are capable of sulfur disproportionation (splitting one compound into two different compounds, in this case an electron donor and an electron acceptor) using elemental sulfur (S^o), sulfite (SO_3^{2-}), and thiosulfate ($S_2O_3^{2-}$) to produce both hydrogen sulfide (H_2S) and sulfate (SO_4^{2-}).

Energy for Reduction

All sulfate-reducing organisms are strict anaerobes. Because sulfate is energetically stable, before it can be metabolized it must first be activated by adenylation to form APS (adenosine 5'-phosphosulfate) thereby consuming ATP. The APS is then reduced by the enzyme APS reductase to form sulfite (SO_3^{2-}) and AMP. In organisms that use carbon compounds as electron donors, the ATP consumed is accounted for by fermentation of the carbon substrate. The hydrogen produced during fermentation is actually what drives respiration during sulfate reduction.

Acetogenesis – Carbon Dioxide as Electron Acceptor

Acetogenesis is a type of microbial metabolism that uses hydrogen (H_2) as an electron donor and carbon dioxide (CO_2) as an electron acceptor to produce acetate, the same electron donors and acceptors used in methanogenesis. Bacteria that can autotrophically synthesize acetate are called homoacetogens. Carbon dioxide reduction in all homoacetogens occurs by the acetyl-CoA pathway. This pathway is also used for carbon fixation by autotrophic sulfate-reducing bacteria and hydrogenotrophic methanogens. Often homoacetogens can also be fermentative, using the hydrogen and carbon dioxide produced as a result of fermentation to produce acetate, which is secreted as an end product.

Other Inorganic Electron Acceptors

Ferric iron (Fe^{3+}) is a widespread anaerobic terminal electron acceptor both for autotrophic and heterotrophic organisms. Electron flow in these organisms is similar to those in electron transport, ending in oxygen or nitrate, except that in ferric iron-reducing organisms the final enzyme in this system is a ferric iron reductase. Model organisms include *Shewanella putrefaciens* and *Geobacter metallireducens*. Since some ferric iron-reducing bacteria (e.g. *G. metallireducens*) can use toxic hydrocarbons such as toluene as a carbon source, there is significant interest in using these organisms as bioremediation agents in ferric iron-rich contaminated aquifers.

Although ferric iron is the most prevalent inorganic electron acceptor, a number of organisms (including the iron-reducing bacteria mentioned above) can use other inorganic ions in anaerobic respiration. While these processes may often be less significant ecologically, they are of considerable interest for bioremediation, especially when heavy metals or radionuclides are used as electron acceptors. Examples include:

- Manganic ion (Mn^{4+}) reduction to manganous ion (Mn^{2+}).
- Selenate (SeO_4^{2-})reduction to selenite (SeO_3^{2-}) and selenite reduction to inorganic selenium (Se^o).
- Arsenate (AsO_4^{3-}) reduction to arsenite (AsO_3^{3-}).
- Uranyl ion ion (UO_2^{2-}) reduction to uranium dioxide (UO_2).

Organic Terminal Electron Acceptors

A number of organisms, instead of using inorganic compounds as terminal electron acceptors, are able to use organic compounds to accept electrons from respiration. Examples include:

- Fumarate reduction to succinate.
- Trimethylamine *N*-oxide (TMAO) reduction to trimethylamine (TMA).
- Dimethyl sulfoxide (DMSO) reduction to Dimethyl sulfide (DMS).
- Reductive dechlorination.

TMAO is a chemical commonly produced by fish, and when reduced to TMA produces a strong odor. DMSO is a common marine and freshwater chemical which is also odiferous when reduced to DMS. Reductive dechlorination is the process by which chlorinated organic compounds are reduced to form their non-chlorinated endproducts. As chlorinated organic compounds are often important (and difficult to degrade) environmental pollutants, reductive dechlorination is an important process in bioremediation.

Chemolithotrophy

Chemolithotrophy is a type of metabolism where energy is obtained from the oxidation of inorganic compounds. Most chemolithotrophic organisms are also autotrophic. There are two major objectives to chemolithotrophy: the generation of energy (ATP) and the generation of reducing power (NADH).

Hydrogen Oxidation

Many organisms are capable of using hydrogen (H_2) as a source of energy. While several mechanisms of anaerobic hydrogen oxidation have been mentioned previously (e.g. sulfate reducing- and acetogenic bacteria), hydrogen can also be used as an energy source aerobically in the knallgas reaction:

$$2H_2 + O_2 \rightarrow 2\ H_2O + \text{energy}$$

In these organisms, hydrogen is oxidized by a membrane-bound hydrogenase causing proton pumping via electron transfer to various quinones and cytochromes. In many organisms, a second cytoplasmic hydrogenase is used to generate reducing power in the form of NADH, which is subsequently used to fix carbon dioxide via the Calvin cycle. Hydrogen-oxidizing organisms, such as *Cupriavidus necator* (formerly *Ralstonia eutropha*), often inhabit oxic-anoxic interfaces in nature to take advantage of the hydrogen produced by anaerobic fermentative organisms while still maintaining a supply of oxygen.

Sulfur Oxidation

Sulfur oxidation involves the oxidation of reduced sulfur compounds (such as sulfide H_2S), inorganic sulfur (S), and thiosulfate ($S_2O_3^{2-}$) to form sulfuric acid (H_2SO_4). A classic example of a sulfur-oxidizing bacterium is *Beggiatoa*, a microbe originally described by Sergei Winogradsky, one of the founders of environmental microbiology. Another example is *Paracoccus*. Generally, the oxidation of sulfide occurs in stages, with inorganic sulfur being stored either inside or outside of the cell until needed. This two step process occurs because energetically sulfide is a better electron donor than inorganic sulfur or thiosulfate, allowing for a greater number of protons to be translocated across the membrane. Sulfur-oxidizing organisms generate reducing power for carbon dioxide fixation via the Calvin cycle using reverse electron flow, an energy-requiring process that pushes the electrons against their thermodynamic gradient to produce NADH. Biochemically, reduced sulfur compounds are converted to sulfite (SO_3^{2-}) and subsequently converted to sulfate (SO_4^{2-}) by the enzyme sulfite oxidase. Some organisms, however, accomplish the same oxidation using a reversal of the APS reductase system used by sulfate-reducing bacteria. In all cases the energy liberated is transferred to the electron transport chain for ATP and NADH production. In addition to aerobic sulfur oxidation, some organisms (e.g. *Thiobacillus denitrificans*) use nitrate (NO_3^-) as a terminal electron acceptor and therefore grow anaerobically.

Ferrous Iron (Fe^{2+}) Oxidation

Ferrous iron is a soluble form of iron that is stable at extremely low pHs or under anaerobic conditions. Under aerobic, moderate pH conditions ferrous iron is oxidized spontaneously to the ferric (Fe^{3+}) form and is hydrolyzed abiotically to insoluble ferric hydroxide ($Fe(OH)_3$). There are three distinct types of ferrous iron-oxidizing microbes. The first are acidophiles, such as the bacteria *Acidithiobacillus ferrooxidans* and *Leptospirillum ferrooxidans,* as well as the archaeon *Ferroplasma*. These microbes oxidize iron in environments that have a very low pH and are important in acid mine drainage. The second type of microbes oxidize ferrous iron at near-neutral pH. These micro-organisms (for example *Gallionella ferruginea, Leptothrix ochracea,* or *Mariprofundus ferrooxydans*) live at the oxic-anoxic interfaces and are microaerophiles. The third type of iron-oxidizing microbes are anaerobic photosynthetic bacteria such as Rhodopseudomonas, which use ferrous iron to produce NADH for autotrophic carbon dioxide fixation. Biochemically, aerobic iron oxidation is a very energetically poor process which therefore requires large amounts of iron to be oxidized by the enzyme rusticyanin to facilitate the formation of proton motive force. Like sulfur oxidation, reverse electron flow must be used to form the NADH used for carbon dioxide fixation via the Calvin cycle.

Nitrification

Nitrification is the process by which ammonia (NH_3) is converted to nitrate (NO_3^-). Nitrification is actually the net result of two distinct processes: oxidation of ammonia to nitrite (NO_2^-) by nitrosifying bacteria (e.g. *Nitrosomonas*) and oxidation of nitrite to nitrate by the nitrite-oxidizing bacteria (e.g. *Nitrobacter*). Both of these processes are extremely energetically poor leading to very slow growth rates for both types of organisms. Biochemically, ammonia oxidation occurs by the stepwise oxidation of ammonia to hydroxylamine (NH_2OH) by the enzyme ammonia monooxygenase in the cytoplasm, followed by the oxidation of hydroxylamine to nitrite by the enzyme hydroxylamine oxidoreductase in the periplasm.

Electron and proton cycling are very complex but as a net result only one proton is translocated across the membrane per molecule of ammonia oxidized. Nitrite oxidation is much simpler, with nitrite being oxidized by the enzyme nitrite oxidoreductase coupled to proton translocation by a very short electron transport chain, again leading to very low growth rates for these organisms. Oxygen is required in both ammonia and nitrite oxidation, meaning that both nitrosifying and nitrite-oxidizing bacteria are aerobes. As in sulfur and iron oxidation, NADH for carbon dioxide fixation using the Calvin cycle is generated by reverse electron flow, thereby placing a further metabolic burden on an already energy-poor process.

In 2015, two groups independently showed the microbial genus *Nitrospira* is capable of complete nitrification (Comammox).

Anammox

Anammox stands for anaerobic ammonia oxidation and the organisms responsible were relatively recently discovered, in the late 1990s. This form of metabolism occurs in members of the Planctomycetes (e.g. Candidatus *Brocadia anammoxidans*) and involves the coupling of ammonia oxidation to nitrite reduction. As oxygen is not required for this process, these organisms are strict anaerobes. Amazingly, hydrazine (N_2H_4 – rocket fuel) is produced as an intermediate during anammox metabolism. To deal with the high toxicity of hydrazine, anammox bacteria contain a hydrazine-containing intracellular organelle called the anammoxasome, surrounded by highly compact (and unusual) ladderane lipid membrane. These lipids are unique in nature, as is the use of hydrazine as a metabolic intermediate. Anammox organisms are autotrophs although the mechanism for carbon dioxide fixation is unclear. Because of this property, these organisms could be used to remove nitrogen in industrial wastewater treatment processes. Anammox has also been shown to have widespread occurrence in anaerobic aquatic systems and has been speculated to account for approximately 50% of nitrogen gas production in the ocean.

Phototrophy

Many microbes (phototrophs) are capable of using light as a source of energy to produce ATP and organic compounds such as carbohydrates, lipids, and proteins. Of these, algae are particularly significant because they are oxygenic, using water as an electron donor for electron transfer during photosynthesis. Phototrophic bacteria are found in the phyla Cyanobacteria, Chlorobi, Proteobacteria, Chloroflexi, and Firmicutes. Along with plants these microbes are responsible for all biological generation of oxygen gas on Earth. Because chloroplasts were derived from a lineage of the Cyanobacteria, the general principles of metabolism in these endosymbionts can also be applied to chloroplasts. In addition to oxygenic photosynthesis, many bacteria can also photosynthesize anaerobically, typically using sulfide (H_2S) as an electron donor to produce sulfate. Inorganic sulfur (S_0), thiosulfate ($S_2O_3^{2-}$) and ferrous iron (Fe^{2+}) can also be used by some organisms. Phylogenetically, all oxygenic photosynthetic bacteria are Cyanobacteria, while anoxygenic photosynthetic bacteria belong to the purple bacteria (Proteobacteria), Green sulfur bacteria (e.g. Chlorobium), Green non-sulfur bacteria (e.g. Chloroflexus), or the heliobacteria (Low %G+C Gram positives). In addition to these organisms, some microbes (e.g. the Archaeon *Halobacterium* or the bacterium *Roseobacter*, among others) can utilize light to produce energy using the enzyme bacteriorhodopsin, a light-driven proton pump. However, there are no known Archaea that carry out photosynthesis.

As befits the large diversity of photosynthetic bacteria, there are many different mechanisms by which light is converted into energy for metabolism. All photosynthetic organisms locate their photosynthetic reaction centers within a membrane, which may be invaginations of the cytoplasmic membrane (Proteobacteria), thylakoid membranes (Cyanobacteria), specialized antenna structures called chlorosomes (Green sulfur and non-sulfur bacteria), or the cytoplasmic membrane itself (heliobacteria). Different photosynthetic bacteria also contain different photosynthetic pigments, such as chlorophylls and carotenoids, allowing them to take advantage of different portions of the electromagnetic spectrum and thereby inhabit different niches. Some groups of organisms contain more specialized light-harvesting structures (e.g. phycobilisomes in Cyanobacteria and chlorosomes in Green sulfur and non-sulfur bacteria), allowing for increased efficiency in light utilization.

Biochemically, anoxygenic photosynthesis is very different from oxygenic photosynthesis. Cyanobacteria (and by extension, chloroplasts) use the Z scheme of electron flow in which electrons eventually are used to form NADH. Two different reaction centers (photosystems) are used and proton motive force is generated both by using cyclic electron flow and the quinone pool. In anoxygenic photosynthetic bacteria, electron flow is cyclic, with all electrons used in photosynthesis eventually being transferred back to the single reaction center. A proton motive force is generated using only the quinone pool. In heliobacteria, Green sulfur, and Green non-sulfur bacteria, NADH is formed using the protein ferredoxin, an energetically favorable reaction. In purple bacteria, NADH is formed by reverse electron flow due to the lower chemical potential of this reaction center. In all cases, however, a proton motive force is generated and used to drive ATP production via an ATPase.

Most photosynthetic microbes are autotrophic, fixing carbon dioxide via the Calvin cycle. Some photosynthetic bacteria (e.g. Chloroflexus) are photoheterotrophs, meaning that they use organic carbon compounds as a carbon source for growth. Some photosynthetic organisms also fix nitrogen.

Nitrogen Fixation

Nitrogen is an element required for growth by all biological systems. While extremely common (80% by volume) in the atmosphere, dinitrogen gas (N_2) is generally biologically inaccessible due to its high activation energy. Throughout all of nature, only specialized bacteria and Archaea are capable of nitrogen fixation, converting dinitrogen gas into ammonia (NH_3), which is easily assimilated by all organisms. These prokaryotes, therefore, are very important ecologically and are often essential for the survival of entire ecosystems. This is especially true in the ocean, where nitrogen-fixing cyanobacteria are often the only sources of fixed nitrogen, and in soils, where specialized symbioses exist between legumes and their nitrogen-fixing partners to provide the nitrogen needed by these plants for growth.

Nitrogen fixation can be found distributed throughout nearly all bacterial lineages and physiological classes but is not a universal property. Because the enzyme nitrogenase, responsible for nitrogen fixation, is very sensitive to oxygen which will inhibit it irreversibly, all nitrogen-fixing organisms must possess some mechanism to keep the concentration of oxygen low. Examples include:

- Heterocyst formation (cyanobacteria e.g. *Anabaena*) where one cell does not photosynthesize but instead fixes nitrogen for its neighbors which in turn provide it with energy.
- Root nodule symbioses (e.g. *Rhizobium*) with plants that supply oxygen to the bacteria bound to molecules of leghaemoglobin.
- Anaerobic lifestyle (e.g. *Clostridium pasteurianum*).
- Very fast metabolism (e.g. *Azotobacter vinelandii*).

The production and activity of nitrogenases is very highly regulated, both because nitrogen fixation is an extremely energetically expensive process (16–24 ATP are used per N_2 fixed) and due to the extreme sensitivity of the nitrogenase to oxygen.

ATP in Metabolism

Adenosine triphosphate or ATP is often called the energy currency of the cell because this molecule plays a key role in metabolism, particularly in energy transfer within cells. The molecule acts to couple the energy of exergonic and endergonic processes, making energetically unfavorable chemical reactions able to proceed.

Metabolic Reactions Involving ATP

Adenosine triphosphate is used to transport chemical energy in many important processes, including:

- Aerobic respiration (glycolysis and the citric acid cycle).
- Fermentation.
- Cellular division.
- Photophosphorylation.
- Motility (e.g., shortening of myosin and actin filament cross-bridges as well as cytoskeleton construction).
- Exocytosis and endocytosis.
- Photosynthesis.
- Protein synthesis.

In addition to metabolic functions, ATP is involved in signal transduction. It is believed to be the neurotransmitter responsible for the sensation of taste. The human central and peripheral nervous system, in particular, relies on ATP signaling. ATP is also added to nucleic acids during transcription.

ATP is continuously recycled, rather than expended. It's converted back into precursor molecules, so it can be used again and again. In human beings, for example, the amount of ATP recycled daily is about the same as body weight, even though the average human being only has about 250 grams of ATP. Another way to look at it is that a single molecule of ATP gets recycled 500-700 times every day. At any moment in time, the amount of ATP plus ADP is fairly constant. This is important since ATP is not a molecule that can be stored for later use.

ATP may be produced from simple and complex sugars as well as from lipids via redox reactions. For this to occur, the carbohydrates must first be broken down into simple sugars, while the lipids must be broken into fatty acids and glycerol. However, ATP production is highly regulated. Its production is controlled via substrate concentration, feedback mechanisms, and allosteric hindrance.

ATP Structure

As indicated by the molecular name, adenosine triphosphate consists of three phosphate groups (tri-prefix before phosphate) connected to adenosine. Adenosine is made by attaching the 9' nitrogen atom of the purine base adenine to the 1' carbon of the pentose sugar ribose. The phosphate groups are attached connecting and oxygen from a phosphate to the 5' carbon of the ribose. Starting with the group closest to the ribose sugar, the phosphate groups are named alpha (α), beta (β), and gamma (γ). Removing a phosphate group results in adenosine diphosphate (ADP) and removing two groups produces adenosine monophosphate (AMP).

How ATP Produces Energy

The key to energy production lies with the phosphate groups. Breaking the phosphate bond is an exothermic reaction. So, when ATP loses one or two phosphate groups, energy is released. More energy is released breaking the first phosphate bond than the second.

$$ATP + H_2O \rightarrow ADP + Pi + Energy\ (\Delta G = -30.5\ kJ.mol^{-1})$$

$$ATP + H_2O \rightarrow AMP + PPi + Energy\ (\Delta G = -45.6\ kJ.mol^{-1})$$

The energy that is released is coupled to an endothermic (thermodynamically unfavorable) reaction in order to give it the activation energy needed to proceed.

Basal Metabolic Rate

Basal metabolic rate (BMR) is the rate of energy expenditure per unit time by endothermic animals at rest. It is reported in energy units per unit time ranging from watt (joule/second) to ml O_2/min or joule per hour per kg body mass J/(h·kg). Proper measurement requires a strict set of criteria be met. These criteria include being in a physically and psychologically undisturbed state, in a thermally neutral environment, while in the post-absorptive state (i.e., not actively digesting food). In bradymetabolic animals, such as fish and reptiles, the equivalent term standard metabolic rate (SMR) is used. It follows the same criteria as BMR, but requires the documentation of the temperature at which the metabolic rate was measured. This makes BMR a variant of standard metabolic rate measurement that excludes the temperature data, a practice that has led to problems in defining "standard" rates of metabolism for many mammals.

Metabolism comprises the processes that the body needs to function. Basal metabolic rate is the amount of energy per unit time that a person needs to keep the body functioning at rest. Some of those processes are breathing, blood circulation, controlling body temperature, cell growth, brain and nerve function, and contraction of muscles. Basal metabolic rate (BMR) affects the rate that a person burns calories and ultimately whether that individual maintains, gains, or loses weight. The basal metabolic rate accounts for about 60 to 75% of the daily calorie expenditure by individuals. It is influenced by several factors. BMR typically declines by 1–2% per decade after age 20, mostly due to loss of fat-free mass, although the variability between individuals is high.

The body's generation of heat is known as thermogenesis and it can be measured to determine the amount of energy expended. BMR generally decreases with age, and with the decrease in lean body mass (as may happen with aging). Increasing muscle mass has the effect of increasing BMR. Aerobic (resistance) fitness level, a product of cardiovascular exercise, while previously thought to have effect on BMR, has been shown in the 1990s not to correlate with BMR when adjusted for fat-free body mass. But anaerobic exercise does increase resting energy consumption. Illness, previously consumed food and beverages, environmental temperature, and stress levels can affect one's overall energy expenditure as well as one's BMR.

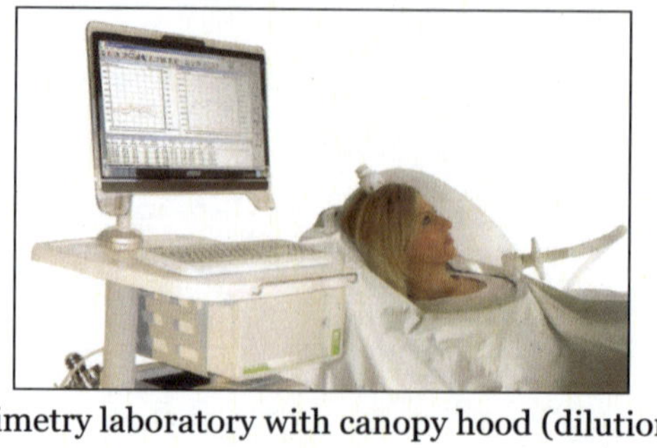

Indirect calorimetry laboratory with canopy hood (dilution technique).

BMR is measured under very restrictive circumstances when a person is awake. An accurate BMR measurement requires that the person's sympathetic nervous system not be stimulated, a condition which requires complete rest. A more common measurement, which uses less strict criteria, is resting metabolic rate (RMR).

BMR may be measured by gas analysis through either direct or indirect calorimetry, though a rough estimation can be acquired through an equation using age, sex, height, and weight. Studies of energy metabolism using both methods provide convincing evidence for the validity of the respiratory quotient (RQ), which measures the inherent composition and utilization of carbohydrates, fats and proteins as they are converted to energy substrate units that can be used by the body as energy.

Phenotypic Flexibility

BMR is a flexible trait (it can be reversibly adjusted within individuals), with, for example, lower temperatures generally resulting in higher basal metabolic rates for both birds and rodents. There are two models to explain how BMR changes in response to temperature: the variable maximum model (VMM) and variable fraction model (VFM). The VMM states that the summit metabolism (or the maximum metabolic rate in response to the cold) increases during the winter, and that the sustained metabolism (or themetabolic rate that can be indefinitely sustained) remains a constant fraction of the former. The VFM says that the summit metabolism does not change, but that the sustained metabolism is a larger fraction of it. The VMM is supported in mammals, and, when using whole-body rates, passerine birds. The VFM is supported in studies of passerine birds using mass-specific metabolic rates (or metabolic rates per unit of mass). This latter measurement has been criticized by Eric Liknes, Sarah Scott, and David Swanson, who say that mass-specific metabolic rates are inconsistent seasonally.

In addition to adjusting to temperature, BMR also may adjust before annual migration cycles. The red knot (ssp. *islandica*) increases its BMR by about 40% before migrating northward. This is because of the energetic demand of long-distance flights. The increase is likely primarily due to increased mass in organs related to flight. The end destination of migrants affects their BMR: yellow-rumped warblers migrating northward were found to have a 31% higher BMR than those migrating southward.

In humans, BMR is directly proportional to a person's lean body mass. In other words, the more lean body mass a person has, the higher their BMR; but BMR is also affected by acute illnesses and increases with conditions like burns, fractures, infections, fevers, etc. In menstruating females, BMR varies to some extent with the phases of their menstrual cycle. Due to the increase in progesterone, BMR rises at the start of the luteal phase and stays at its highest until this phase ends. There are different findings in research how much of an increase usually occurs. Small sample, early studies, found various figures, such as; a 6% higher postovulatory sleep metabolism, a 7% to 15% higher 24 hour expenditure following ovulation, and an increase and a luteal phase BMR increase by up to 12%. A study by the American Society of Clinical Nutrition found that an experimental group of female volunteers had an 11.5% average increase in 24 hour energy expenditure in the two weeks following ovulation, with a range of 8% to 16%. This group was measured via simultaneously direct and indirect calorimetry and had standardized daily meals and sedentary schedule in order to prevent the increase from being manipulated by change in food intake or activity level. A 2011 study conducted by the Mandya Institute of Medical Sciences found that during a woman's follicular phase and menstrual cycle is no significant difference in BMR, however the calories burned per hour is significantly higher, up to 18%, during the luteal phase. Increased state anxiety (stress level) also temporarily increased BMR.

Physiology

The early work of the scientists J. Arthur Harris and Francis G. Benedict showed that approximate values for BMR could be derived using body surface area (computed from height and weight), age, and sex, along with the oxygen and carbon dioxide measures taken from calorimetry. Studies also showed that by eliminating the sex differences that occur with the accumulation of adipose tissue by expressing metabolic rate per unit of "fat-free" or lean body mass, the values between sexes for basal metabolism are essentially the same. Exercise physiology textbooks have tables to show the conversion of height and body surface area as they relate to weight and basal metabolic values.

The primary organ responsible for regulating metabolism is the hypothalamus. The hypothalamus is located on the diencephalon and forms the floor and part of the lateral walls of the third ventricle of the cerebrum. The chief functions of the hypothalamus are:

1. Control and integration of activities of the autonomic nervous system (ANS):
    - The ANS regulates contraction of smooth muscle and cardiac muscle, along with secretions of many endocrine organs such as the thyroid gland (associated with many metabolic disorders).
    - Through the ANS, the hypothalamus is the main regulator of visceral activities, such as heart rate, movement of food through the gastrointestinal tract, and contraction of the urinary bladder.
2. Production and regulation of feelings of rage and aggression.
3. Regulation of body temperature.
4. Regulation of food intake, through two centers:
    - The feeding center or hunger center is responsible for the sensations that cause us to seek food. When sufficient food or substrates have been received and leptin is high, then the satiety center is stimulated and sends impulses

that inhibit the feeding center. When insufficient food is present in the stomach and ghrelin levels are high, receptors in the hypothalamus initiate the sense of hunger.

- The thirst center operates similarly when certain cells in the hypothalamus are stimulated by the rising osmotic pressure of the extracellular fluid. If thirst is satisfied, osmotic pressure decreases.

All of these functions taken together form a survival mechanism that causes us to sustain the body processes that BMR measures.

BMR Estimation Formulas

Several equations to predict the number of calories required by humans have been published from the early 20th–21st centuries. In each of the formulas below:

- P is total heat production at complete rest,
- m is mass (kg),
- h is height (cm), and
- a is age (years).

The Original Harris-Benedict Equation

Historically, the most notable formula was the Harris–Benedict equation, which was published in 1919.

- For men, $P = \left(\frac{13.7516m}{1\,\text{kg}} + \frac{5.0033h}{1\,\text{cm}} - \frac{6.7550a}{1\,\text{year}} + 66.4730 \right) \frac{\text{kcal}}{\text{day}}$.
- For women, $P = \left(\frac{9.5634m}{1\,\text{kg}} + \frac{1.8496h}{1\,\text{cm}} - \frac{4.6756a}{1\,\text{year}} + 655.0955 \right) \frac{\text{kcal}}{\text{day}}$.

The difference in BMR for men and women is mainly due to differences in body weight. For example, a 55 year-old woman weighing 130 lb (59 kg) and 5 feet 6 inches (168 cm) tall would have a BMR of 1272 kcal per day.

The Revised Harris-Benedict Equation

In 1984, the original Harris-Benedict equations were revised using new data. In comparisons with actual expenditure, the revised equations were found to be more accurate.

- For men, $P = \left(\frac{13.397m}{1\,\text{kg}} + \frac{4.799h}{1\,\text{cm}} - \frac{5.677a}{1\,\text{year}} + 88.362 \right) \frac{\text{kcal}}{\text{day}}$.

- For women, $P = \left(\frac{9.247m}{1\,\text{kg}} + \frac{3.098h}{1\,\text{cm}} - \frac{4.330a}{1\,\text{year}} + 447.593 \right) \frac{\text{kcal}}{\text{day}}$.

It was the best prediction equation until 1990, when Mifflin *et al.* introduced the equation:

The Mifflin St Jeor Equation

- $P = \left(\frac{10.0m}{1\,\text{kg}} + \frac{6.25h}{1\,\text{cm}} - \frac{5.0a}{1\,\text{year}} + s \right) \frac{\text{kcal}}{\text{day}}$, where s is +5 for males and −161 for females.

According to this formula, the woman in the example above has a BMR of 1204 kcal per day. During the last 100 years, lifestyles have changed and Frankenfield *et al.* showed it to be about 5% more accurate.

These formulas are based on body weight, which does not take into account the difference in metabolic activity between lean body mass and body fat. Other formulas exist which take into account lean body mass, two of which are the Katch-McArdle formula, and Cunningham formula.

The Katch-McArdle Formula

The Katch-McArdle formula is used to predict Resting Daily Energy Expenditure (RDEE). The Cunningham formula is commonly cited to predict RMR instead of BMR; however, the formulas provided by Katch-McArdle and Cunningham are the same.

- $P = 370 + (21.6 \cdot \ell)$.

where ℓ is the lean body mass (*LBM* in kg)

- $\ell = m\left(1 - \frac{f}{100}\right)$.

where f is the body fat percentage. According to this formula, if the woman in the example has a body fat percentage of 30%, her Resting Daily Energy Expenditure (the authors use the term of basal and resting metabolism interchangeably) would be 1262 kcal per day.

Causes of Individual Differences in BMR

The basic metabolic rate varies between individuals. One study of 150 adults representative of the population in Scotland reported basal metabolic rates from as low as 1027 kcal per day (4301 kJ/day) to as high as 2499 kcal/day (10455 kJ/day); with a mean BMR of 1500 kcal/day (6279 kJ/day). Statistically, the researchers calculated that 62.3% of this variation was explained by differences in fat free mass. Other factors explaining the variation included fat mass (6.7%), age (1.7%), and experimental error including within-subject difference (2%). The rest of the variation (26.7%) was unexplained. This remaining difference was not explained by sex nor by differing tissue size of highly energetic organs such as the brain.

Differences in BMR have been observed when comparing subjects with *the same* lean body mass. In one study, when comparing individuals with the same lean body mass, the top 5% of BMRs are 1.28–1.32 times the lowest 5% BMR. Additionally, this study reports a case where two individuals with the same lean body mass of 43 kg had BMRs of 1075 kcal/day (4.5 MJ/day) and 1790 kcal/day (7.5 MJ/day). This difference of 715 kcal/day (67%) is equivalent to one of the individuals completing a 10 kilometer run every day. However, this study did not account for the sex, height, fasting-state, or body fat percentage of the subjects.

Biochemistry

Energy Expenditure Breakdown	
Liver	27%
Brain	19%
Skeletal Muscle	18%
Kidneys	10%
Heart	7%
Other organs	19%

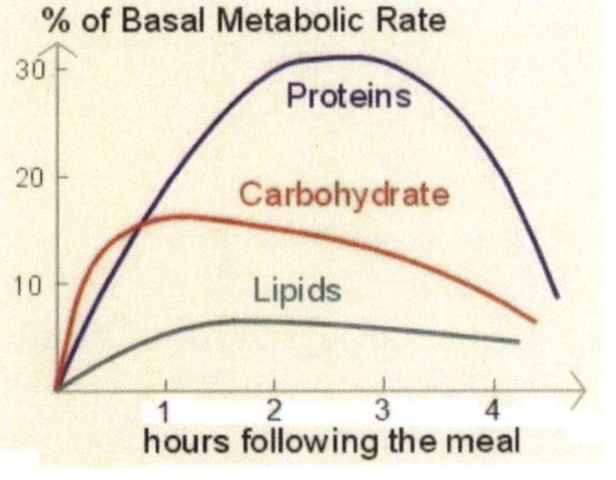

Postprandial thermogenesis increases in basal metabolic rate occur at different degrees depending on consumed food composition.

About 70% of a human's total energy expenditure is due to the basal life processes taking place in the organs of the body. About 20% of one's energy expenditure comes from physical activity and another 10% from thermogenesis, or digestion of food (*postprandial thermogenesis*). All of these processes require an intake of oxygen along with coenzymes to provide energy for survival (usually from macronutrients like carbohydrates, fats, and proteins) and expel carbon dioxide, due to processing by the Krebs cycle.

For the BMR, most of the energy is consumed in maintaining fluid levels in tissues through osmoregulation, and only about one-tenth is consumed for mechanical work, such as digestion, heartbeat, and breathing.

What enables the Krebs cycle to perform metabolic changes to fats, carbohydrates, and proteins is energy, which can be defined as the ability or capacity to do work. The breakdown of large molecules into smaller molecules—associated with release of energy—is catabolism. The building up process is termed anabolism. The breakdown of proteins into amino acids is an example of catabolism, while the formation of proteins from amino acids is an anabolic process.

Exergonic reactions are energy-releasing reactions and are generally catabolic. Endergonic reactions require energy and include anabolic reactions and the contraction of muscle. Metabolism is the total of all catabolic, exergonic, anabolic, endergonic reactions.

Adenosine Triphosphate (ATP) is the intermediate molecule that drives the exergonic transfer of energy to switch to endergonic anabolic reactions used in muscle contraction. This is what causes muscles to work which can require a breakdown, and also to build in the rest period, which occurs during the strengthening phase associated with muscular contraction. ATP is composed of adenine, a nitrogen containing base, ribose, a five carbon sugar (collectively called adenosine), and three phosphate groups. ATP is a high energy molecule because it stores large amounts of energy in the chemical bonds of the two terminal phosphate groups. The breaking of these chemical bonds in the Krebs Cycle provides the energy needed for muscular contraction.

Glucose

Because the ratio of hydrogen to oxygen atoms in all carbohydrates is always the same as that in water—that is, 2 to 1—all of the oxygen consumed by the cells is used to oxidize the carbon in the carbohydrate molecule to form carbon dioxide. Consequently, during the complete oxidation of a glucose molecule, six molecules of carbon dioxide and six molecules of water are produced and six molecules of oxygen are consumed.

The overall equation for this reaction is:

$$C_6H_{12}O_6 + 6\,O_2 \rightarrow 6\,CO_2 + 6\,H_2O.$$

38 ATP molecules

Because the gas exchange in this reaction is equal, the respiratory quotient (R.Q.) for carbohydrate is unity or 1.0:

$$R.Q. = 6\,CO_2/6\,O_2 = 1.0.$$

Fats

The chemical composition for fats differs from that of carbohydrates in that fats contain considerably fewer oxygen atoms in proportion to atoms of carbon and hydrogen. When listed on nutritional information tables, fats are generally divided into six categories: total fats, saturated fatty acid, polyunsaturated fatty acid, monounsaturated fatty acid, dietary cholesterol, and trans fatty acid. From a basal metabolic or resting metabolic perspective, more energy is needed to burn a saturated fatty acid than an unsaturated fatty acid. The fatty acid molecule is broken down and categorized based on the number of carbon atoms in its molecular structure. The chemical equation for metabolism of the twelve to sixteen carbon atoms in a saturated fatty acid molecule shows the difference between metabolism of carbohydrates and fatty acids. Palmitic acid is a commonly studied example of the saturated fatty acid molecule.

The overall equation for the substrate utilization of palmitic acid is:

$$C_{16}H_{32}O_2 + 23\ O_2 \rightarrow 16\ CO_2 + 16\ H_2O.$$

Thus the R.Q. for palmitic acid is 0.696:

$$R.Q. = 16\ CO_2 / 23\ O_2 = 0.696.$$

Proteins

Proteins are composed of carbon, hydrogen, oxygen, and nitrogen arranged in a variety of ways to form a large combination of amino acids. Unlike fat the body has no storage deposits of protein. All of it is contained in the body as important parts of tissues, blood hormones, and enzymes. The structural components of the body that contain these amino acids are continually undergoing a process of breakdown and replacement. The respiratory quotient for protein metabolism can be demonstrated by the chemical equation for oxidation of albumin:

$$C_{72}H_{112}N_{18}O_{22}S + 77\ O_2 \rightarrow 63\ CO_2 + 38\ H_2O + SO_3 + 9\ CO(NH_2)_2$$

The R.Q. for albumin is $63\ CO_2 / 77\ O_2 = 0.818$.

The reason this is important in the process of understanding protein metabolism is that the body can blend the three macronutrients and based on the mitochondrial density, a preferred ratio can be established which determines how much fuel is utilized in which packets for work accomplished by the muscles. Protein catabolism (breakdown) has been estimated to supply 10% to 15% of the total energy requirement during a two-hour aerobic training session. This process could severely degrade the protein structures needed to maintain survival such as contractile properties of proteins in the heart, cellular mitochondria, myoglobin storage, and metabolic enzymes within muscles.

The oxidative system (aerobic) is the primary source of ATP supplied to the body at rest and during low intensity activities and uses primarily carbohydrates and fats as substrates. Protein is not normally metabolized significantly, except during long term starvation and long bouts of exercise (greater than 90 minutes). At rest approximately 70% of the ATP produced is derived from fats and 30% from carbohydrates. Following the onset of activity, as the intensity of the exercise increases, there is a shift in substrate preference from fats to carbohydrates. During high intensity aerobic exercise, almost 100% of the energy is derived from carbohydrates, if an adequate supply is available.

Aerobic vs. Anaerobic Exercise

Studies published in 1992 and 1997 indicate that the level of aerobic fitness of an individual does not have any correlation with the level of resting metabolism. Both studies find that aerobic fitness levels do not improve the predictive power of fat free mass for resting metabolic rate. When you consider time commitments against health benefits, AT is the optimal mode of exercise for reducing fat mass and body mass as a primary consideration, RT is good as a secondary factor when aging and lean mass are a concern. RT causes injuries at a much higher rate than AT. Compared to RT, it was found that AET resulted in a significantly more pronounced reduction of body weight by enhancing the cardiovascular system which is what is the principle factor in metabolic utilization of fat substrates. RT if time is available is also helpful in post exercise metabolism, but it is an adjunctive factor because the body needs to heal sufficiently between RT episodes, whereas with AET, the body can accept this every day. RMR, and BMR are measurements of daily consumption of calories. The majority of studies that are published on this topic look at aerobic exercise because of its efficacy for health and weight management.

Anaerobic exercise, such as weight lifting, builds additional muscle mass. Muscle contributes to the fat-free mass of an individual and therefore effective results from anaerobic exercise will increase BMR. However, the actual effect on BMR is controversial and difficult to enumerate. Various studies suggest that the resting metabolic rate of trained muscle is around 55kJ per kilogram, per day. Even a substantial increase in muscle mass, say 5 kg, would make only a minor impact on BMR.

Longevity

In 1926, Raymond Pearl proposed that longevity varies inversely with basal metabolic rate (the "rate of living hypothesis"). Support for this hypothesis comes from the fact that mammals with larger body size have longer maximum life spans (large animals do have higher total metabolic rates, but the metabolic rate at the cellular level is much lower, and the breathing rate and heartbeat are slower in larger animals) and the fact that the longevity of fruit flies varies inversely with ambient temperature. Additionally, the life span of houseflies can be extended by preventing physical activity. This theory has been bolstered by several new studies linking lower basal metabolic rate to increased life expectancy, across the animal kingdom—including humans. Calorie restriction and reduced thyroid hormone levels, both of which decrease the metabolic rate, have been associated with higher longevity in animals.

However, the ratio of total daily energy expenditure to resting metabolic rate can vary between 1.6 and 8.0 between species of mammals. Animals also vary in the degree of coupling between oxidative phosphorylation and ATP production, the amount of saturated fat in mitochondrial membranes, the amount of DNA repair, and many other factors that affect maximum life span.

Organism Longevity and Basal Metabolic Rate

In allometric scaling, maximum potential life span (MPLS) is directly related to metabolic rate (MR), where MR is the recharge rate of a biomass made up of covalent bonds. That biomass (W) is subjected to deterioration over time from thermodynamic, entropic pressure. Metabolism is essentially understood as redox coupling, and has nothing to do with thermogenesis. Metabolic efficiency (ME) is then expressed as the efficiency of this coupling, a ratio of amperes captured and used by biomass, to the amperes available for that purpose. MR is measured in watts, W is measured in grams. These factors are combined in a power law, an elaboration on Kleiber's law relating MR to W and MPLS, that appears as MR = W^ (4ME-1)/4ME. When ME is 100%, MR = W^3/4; this is popularly known as quarter power scaling, a version of allometric scaling that is premised upon unrealistic estimates of biological efficiency.

The equation reveals that as ME drops below 20%, for $W <$ one gram, MR/MPLS increases so dramatically as to endow W with virtual immortality by 16%. The smaller W is to begin with, the more dramatic is the increase in MR as ME diminishes. All of the cells of an organism fit into this range, i.e., less than one gram, and so this MR will be referred to as BMR.

But the equation reveals that as ME increases over 25%, BMR approaches zero. The equation also shows that for all $W >$ one gram, where W is the organization of all of the BMRs of the organism's structure, but also includes the activity of the structure, as ME increases over 25%, MR/MPLS increases rather than decreases, as it does for BMR. An MR made up of an organization of BMRs will be referred to as an FMR. As ME decreases below 25%, FMR diminishes rather than increases as it does for BMR.

The antagonism between FMR and BMR is what marks the process of aging of biomass W in energetic terms. The ME for the organism is the same as that for the cells, such that the success of the organism's ability to find food (and lower its ME), is key to maintaining the BMR of the cells driven, otherwise, by starvation, to approaching zero; while at the same time a lower ME diminishes the FMR/MPLS of the organism.

Metabolic Pathways

A metabolic pathway is a linked series of chemical reactions occurring within a cell. The reactants, products, and intermediates of an enzymatic reaction are known as metabolites, which are modified by a sequence of chemical reactions catalyzed by enzymes. In most cases of a metabolic pathway, the product of one enzyme acts as the substrate for the next. However, side products are considered waste and removed from the cell. These enzymes often require dietary minerals, vitamins, and other co-factors to function.

Different metabolic pathways function based on the position within a eukaryotic cell and the significance of the pathway in the given compartment of the cell. For instance, the, electron transport chain, and oxidative phosphorylation all take place in the mitochondrial membrane. In contrast, glycolysis, pentose phosphate pathway, and fatty acid biosynthesis all occur in the cytosol of a cell.

There are two types of metabolic pathways that are characterized by their ability to either synthesize molecules with the utilization of energy (anabolic pathway) or break down of complex molecules by releasing energy in the process (catabolic pathway). The two pathways complement each other in that the energy released from one is used up by the other. The degradative process of a catabolic pathway provides the energy required to conduct a biosynthesis of an anabolic pathway. In addition to the two distinct metabolic pathways is the amphibolic pathway, which can be either catabolic or anabolic based on the need for or the availability of energy.

Pathways are required for the maintenance of homeostasis within an organism and the flux of metabolites through a pathway is regulated depending on the needs of the cell and the availability of the substrate. The end product of a pathway may be used immediately, initiate another metabolic pathway or be stored for later use. The metabolism of a cell consists of an elaborate network of interconnected pathways that enable the synthesis and breakdown of molecules (anabolism and catabolism).

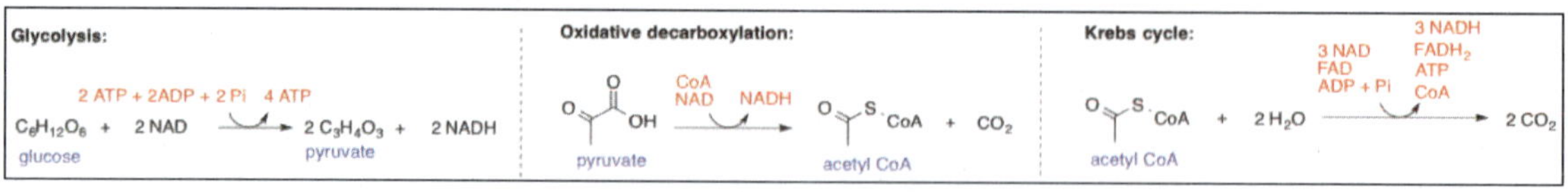

Net Reactions of Common Metabolic Pathways.

Each metabolic pathway consists of a series of biochemical reactions that are connected by their intermediates: the products of one reaction are the substrates for subsequent reactions, and so on. Metabolic pathways are often considered to flow in one direction. Although all chemical reactions are technically reversible, conditions in the cell are often such that it is thermodynamically more favorable for flux to proceed in one direction of a reaction. For example, one pathway may be responsible for the synthesis of a particular amino acid, but the breakdown of that amino acid may occur via a separate and distinct pathway. One example of an exception to this "rule" is the metabolism of glucose. Glycolysis results in the breakdown of glucose, but several reactions in the glycolysis pathway are reversible and participate in the re-synthesis of glucose (gluconeogenesis).

- Glycolysis was the first metabolic pathway discovered:
    - As glucose enters a cell, it is immediately phosphorylated by ATP to glucose 6-phosphate in the irreversible first step.
    - In times of excess lipid or protein energy sources, certain reactions in the glycolysis pathway may run in reverse to produce glucose 6-phosphate, which is then used for storage as glycogen or starch.
- Metabolic pathways are often regulated by feedback inhibition.
- Some metabolic pathways flow in a 'cycle' wherein each component of the cycle is a substrate for the subsequent reaction in the cycle, such as in the Krebs Cycle.
- Anabolic and catabolic pathways in eukaryotes often occur independently of each other, separated either physically by compartmentalization within organelles or separated biochemically by the requirement of different enzymes and co-factors.

Major Metabolic Pathways

Catabolic Pathway (Catabolism)

A catabolic pathway is a series of reactions that bring about a net release of energy in the form of a high energy phosphate bond formed with the energy carriers adenosine diphosphate (ADP) and guanosine diphosphate (GDP) to produce adenosine triphosphate (ATP) and guanosine triphosphate (GTP), respectively. The net reaction is, therefore, thermodynamically favorable, for it results in a lower free energy for the final products. A catabolic pathway is an exergonic system that produces chemical energy in the form of ATP, GTP, NADH, NADPH, FADH2, etc. from energy containing sources such as carbohydrates, fats, and proteins. The end products are often carbon dioxide, water, and ammonia. Coupled with an endergonic reaction of anabolism, the cell can synthesize new macromolecules using the original precursors of the anabolic pathway. An example of a coupled reaction is the phosphorylation of fructose-6-phosphate to form the intermediate fructose-1,6-bisphosphate by the enzyme phosphofructokinase accompanied by the hydrolysis of ATP in the pathway of glycolysis. The resulting chemical reaction within the metabolic pathway is highly thermodynamically favorable and, as a result, irreversible in the cell.

$$Fructose-6-Phosphate+ATP \rightarrow Fructose-1,6-Bisphosphate+ADP.$$

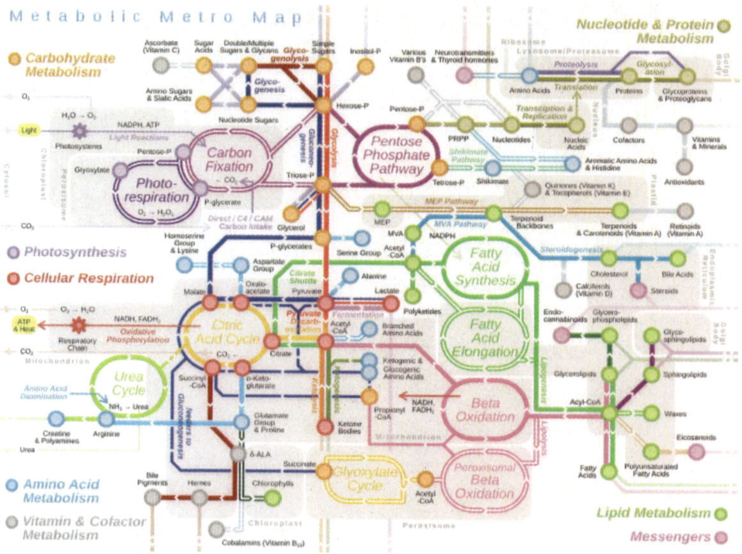

Major metabolic pathways in metro-style map.
Single lines: pathways common to most lifeforms. Double lines: pathways not in humans

- Orange nodes: carbohydrate metabolism.
- Violet nodes: photosynthesis.
- Red nodes: cellular respiration.
- Pink nodes: cell signaling.
- Blue nodes: amino acid metabolism.
- Grey nodes: vitamin and cofactor metabolism.
- Brown nodes: nucleotide and protein metabolism.
- Green nodes: lipid metabolism.

Cellular Respiration

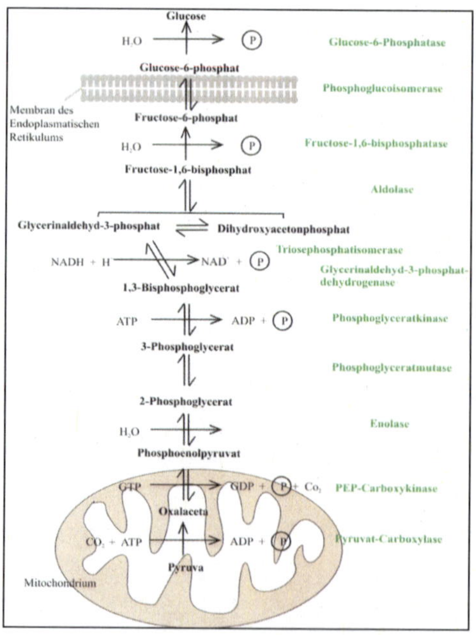

Gluconeogenesis Mechanism.

A core set of energy-producing catabolic pathways occur within all living organisms in some form. These pathways transfer the energy released by breakdown of nutrients into ATP and other small molecules used for energy (e.g. GTP, NADPH, FADH). All cells can perform anaerobic respiration by glycolysis. Additionally, most organisms can perform more efficient aerobic respiration through the citric acid cycle and oxidative phosphorylation. Additionally plants, algae and cyanobacteria are able to use sunlight to anabolically synthesize compounds from non-living matter by photosynthesis.

Anabolic Pathway (Anabolism)

In contrast to catabolic pathways, anabolic pathways require an energy input to construct macromolecules such as polypeptides, nucleic acids, proteins, polysaccharides, and lipids. The isolated reaction of anabolism is unfavorable in a cell due to a positive Gibbs Free Energy ($+\Delta G$). Thus, an input of chemical energy through a coupling with an exergonic reaction is necessary. The coupled reaction of the catabolic pathway affects the thermodynamics of the reaction by lowering the overall activation energy of an anabolic pathway and allowing the reaction to take place. Otherwise, an endergonic reaction is non-spontaneous.

An anabolic pathway is a biosynthetic pathway, meaning that it combines smaller molecules to form larger and more complex ones. An example is the reversed pathway of glycolysis, otherwise known as gluconeogenesis, which occurs in the liver and sometimes in the kidney to maintain proper glucose concentration in the blood and supply the brain and muscle tissues with adequate amount of glucose. Although gluconeogenesis is similar to the reverse pathway of glycolysis, it contains three distinct enzymes from glycolysis that allow the pathway to occur spontaneously. An example of the pathway for gluconeogenesis is illustrated in the image titled “Gluconeogenesis Mechanism”.

Amphibolic Pathway

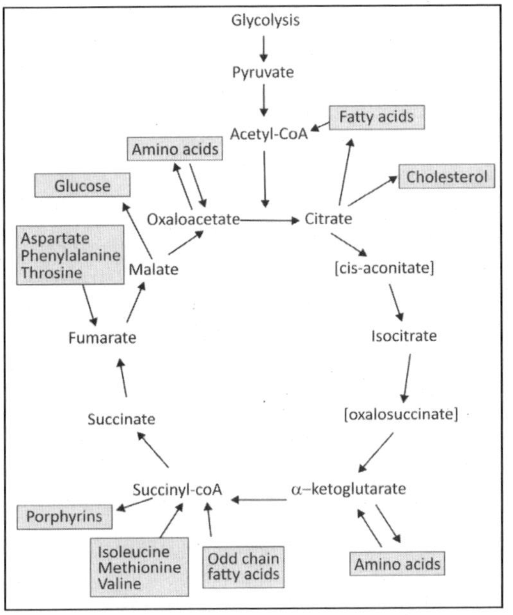

Amphibolic Properties of the Citric Acid Cycle.

An amphibolic pathway is one that can be either catabolic or anabolic based on the availability of or the need for energy. The currency of energy in a biological cell is adenosine triphosphate (ATP), which stores its energy in the phosphoanhydride bonds. The energy is utilized to conduct biosynthesis, facilitate movement, and regulate active transport inside of the cell. Examples of amphibolic pathways are the citric acid cycle and the glyoxylate cycle. These sets of chemical reactions contain both energy producing and utilizing pathways. To the right is an illustration of the amphibolic properties of the TCA cycle.

The glyoxylate shunt pathway is an alternative to the tricarboxylic acid (TCA) cycle, for it redirects the pathway of TCA to prevent full oxidation of carbon compounds, and to preserve high energy carbon sources as future energy sources. This pathway occurs only in plants and bacteria and transpires in the absence of glucose molecules.

Glycolysis

Glycolysis is the metabolic pathway that converts glucose $C_6H_{12}O_6$, into pyruvate, $CH_3COCOO^- + H^+$. The free energy released in this process is used to form the high-energy molecules ATP (adenosine triphosphate) and NADH (reduced nicotinamide adenine dinucleotide). Glycolysis is a sequence of ten enzyme-catalyzed reactions. Most monosaccharides, such as fructose and galactose, can be converted to one of these intermediates. The intermediates may also be directly useful rather than just utilized as steps in the overall reaction. For example, the intermediate dihydroxyacetone phosphate (DHAP) is a source of the glycerol that combines with fatty acids to form fat.

Glycolysis is an oxygen-independent metabolic pathway. The wide occurrence of glycolysis indicates that it is an ancient metabolic pathway. Indeed, the reactions that constitute glycolysis and its parallel pathway, the pentose phosphate pathway, occur metal-catalyzed under the oxygen-free conditions of the Archean oceans, also in the absence of enzymes.

In most organisms, glycolysis occurs in the cytosol. The most common type of glycolysis is the *Embden–Meyerhof–Parnas (EMP pathway)*, which was discovered by Gustav Embden, Otto Meyerhof, and Jakub Karol Parnas. Glycolysis also refers to other pathways, such as the *Entner–Doudoroff pathway* and various heterofermentative and homofermentative pathways. However, the discussion here will be limited to the Embden–Meyerhof–Parnas pathway.

The glycolysis pathway can be separated into two phases:

1. The Preparatory (or Investment) Phase – wherein ATP is consumed.
2. The Pay Off Phase – wherein ATP is produced.

The overall reaction of glycolysis is:

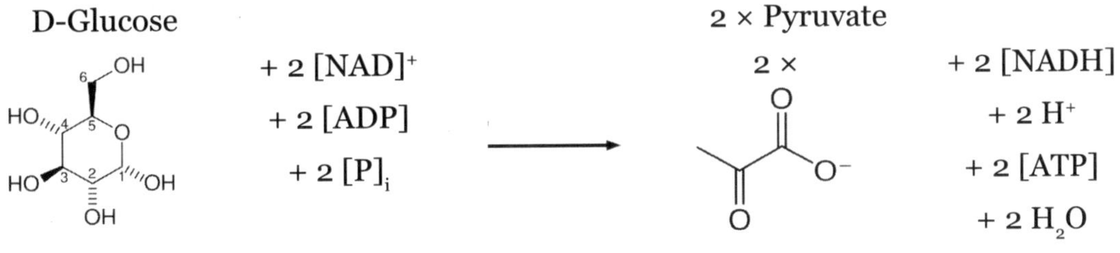

The use of symbols in this equation makes it appear unbalanced with respect to oxygen atoms, hydrogen atoms, and charges. Atom balance is maintained by the two phosphate (P_i) groups:

- Each exists in the form of a hydrogen phosphate anion (HPO_4^{2-}), dissociating to contribute 2 H^+ overall.
- Each liberates an oxygen atom when it binds to an ADP (adenosine diphosphate) molecule, contributing 2 O overall.

Charges are balanced by the difference between ADP and ATP. In the cellular environment, all three hydroxyl groups of ADP dissociate into $-O^-$ and H^+, giving ADP^{3-}, and this ion tends to exist in an ionic bond with Mg^{2+}, giving $ADPMg^-$. ATP behaves identically except that it has four hydroxyl groups, giving $ATPMg^{2-}$. When these differences along with the true charges on the two phosphate groups are considered together, the net charges of −4 on each side are balanced.

For simple fermentations, the metabolism of one molecule of glucose to two molecules of pyruvate has a net yield of two molecules of ATP. Most cells will then carry out further reactions to 'repay' the used NAD^+ and produce a final product of ethanol or lactic acid. Many bacteria use inorganic compounds as hydrogen acceptors to regenerate the NAD^+.

Cells performing aerobic respiration synthesize much more ATP, but not as part of glycolysis. These further aerobic reactions use pyruvate and NADH + H^+ from glycolysis. Eukaryotic aerobic respiration produces approximately 34 additional molecules of ATP for each glucose molecule, however most of these are produced by a vastly different mechanism to the substrate-level phosphorylation in glycolysis.

The lower-energy production, per glucose, of anaerobic respiration relative to aerobic respiration, results in greater flux through the pathway under hypoxic (low-oxygen) conditions, unless alternative sources of anaerobically oxidizable substrates, such as fatty acids, are found.

Post-Glycolysis Processes

The overall process of glycolysis is:

$$\text{Glucose} + 2\ NAD^+ + 2\ ADP + 2\ P_i \rightarrow 2\ \text{Pyruvate} + 2\ NADH + 2\ H^+ + 2\ ATP$$

If glycolysis were to continue indefinitely, all of the NAD^+ would be used up, and glycolysis would stop. To allow glycolysis to continue, organisms must be able to oxidize NADH back to NAD^+. How this is performed depends on which external electron acceptor is available.

Anoxic Regeneration of NAD^+

One method of doing this is to simply have the pyruvate do the oxidation; in this process, pyruvate is converted to lactate (the conjugate base of lactic acid) in a process called lactic acid fermentation:

$$\text{Pyruvate} + \text{NADH} + H^+ \rightarrow \text{Lactate} + \text{NAD}^+$$

This process occurs in the bacteria involved in making yogurt (the lactic acid causes the milk to curdle). This process also occurs in animals under hypoxic (or partially anaerobic) conditions, found, for example, in overworked muscles that are starved of oxygen. In many tissues, this is a cellular last resort for energy; most animal tissue cannot tolerate anaerobic conditions for an extended period of time.

Some organisms, such as yeast, convert NADH back to NAD^+ in a process called ethanol fermentation. In this process, the pyruvate is converted first to acetaldehyde and carbon dioxide, and then to ethanol.

Lactic acid fermentation and ethanol fermentation can occur in the absence of oxygen. This anaerobic fermentation allows many single-cell organisms to use glycolysis as their only energy source.

Anoxic regeneration of NAD^+ is only an effective means of energy production during short, intense exercise in vertebrates, for a period ranging from 10 seconds to 2 minutes during a maximal effort in humans. (At lower exercise intensities it can sustain muscle activity in diving animals, such as seals, whales and other aquatic vertebrates, for very much longer periods of time.) Under these conditions NAD^+ is replenished by NADH donating its electrons to pyruvate to form lactate. This produces 2 ATP molecules per glucose molecule, or about 5% of glucose's energy potential (38 ATP molecules in bacteria). But the speed at which ATP is produced in this manner is about 100 times that of oxidative phosphorylation. The pH in the cytoplasm quickly drops when hydrogen ions accumulate in the muscle, eventually inhibiting the enzymes involved in glycolysis.

The burning sensation in muscles during hard exercise can be attributed to the release of hydrogen ions during the shift to glucose fermentation from glucose oxidation to carbon dioxide and water, when aerobic metabolism can no longer keep pace with the energy demands of the muscles. These hydrogen ions form a part of lactic acid. The body falls back on this less efficient but faster method of producing ATP under low oxygen conditions. This is thought to have been the primary means of energy production in earlier organisms before oxygen reached high concentrations in the atmosphere between 2000 and 2500 million years ago, and thus would represent a more ancient form of energy production than the aerobic replenishment of NAD^+ in cells.

The liver in mammals gets rid of this excess lactate by transforming it back into pyruvate under aerobic conditions.

Fermentation of pyruvate to lactate is sometimes also called “anaerobic glycolysis”, however, glycolysis ends with the production of pyruvate regardless of the presence or absence of oxygen.

In the above two examples of fermentation, NADH is oxidized by transferring two electrons to pyruvate. However, anaerobic bacteria use a wide variety of compounds as the terminal electron acceptors in cellular respiration: nitrogenous compounds, such as nitrates and nitrites; sulfur compounds, such as sulfates, sulfites, sulfur dioxide, and elemental sulfur; carbon dioxide; iron compounds; manganese compounds; cobalt compounds; and uranium compounds.

Aerobic Regeneration of NAD^+ and Disposal of Pyruvate

In aerobic organisms, a complex mechanism has been developed to use the oxygen in air as the final electron acceptor.

- Firstly, the NADH+ H^+ generated by glycolysis has to be transferred to the mitochondrion to be oxidized, and thus to regenerate the NAD^+ necessary for glycolysis to continue. However the inner mitochondrial membrane is impermeable to NADH and NAD^+. Use is therefore made of two “shuttles” to transport the electrons from NADH across the mitochondrial membrane. They are the malate-aspartate shuttle and the glycerol phosphate shuttle. In the former the electrons from NADH are transferred to cytosolic oxaloacetate to form malate. The malate then traverses the inner mitochondrial membrane into the mitochondrial matrix, where it is reoxidized by NAD^+ forming intra-mitochondrial oxaloacetate and NADH. The oxaloacetate is then re-cycled to the cytosol via its conversion to aspartate which is readily transported out of the mitochondrion. In the glycerol phosphate shuttle electrons from cytosolic NADH are transferred to dihydroxyacetone to form glycerol-3-phosphate which readily traverses the outer mitochondrial membrane. Glycerol-3-phosphate is then reoxidized to dihydroxyacetone, donating its electrons to FAD instead of NAD^+. This reaction takes place on the inner mitochondrial membrane, allowing $FADH_2$ to donate its electrons directly to coenzyme Q (ubiquinone) which is part of the electron transport chain which ultimately transfers electrons to molecular oxygen (O_2), with the formation of water, and the release of energy eventually captured in the form of ATP.
- The glycolytic end-product, pyruvate (plus NAD^+) is converted to acetyl-CoA, CO_2 and NADH + H^+ within the mitochondria in a process called pyruvate decarboxylation.

- The resulting acetyl-CoA enters the citric acid cycle (or Krebs Cycle), where the acetyl group of the acetyl-CoA is converted into carbon dioxide by two decarboxylation reactions with the formation of yet more intra-mitochondrial NADH + H^+.
- The intra-mitochondrial NADH + H^+ is oxidized to NAD^+ by the electron transport chain, using oxygen as the final electron acceptor to form water. The energy released during this process is used to create a hydrogen ion (or proton) gradient across the inner membrane of the mitochondrion.
- Finally, the proton gradient is used to produce about 2.5 ATP for every NADH + H^+ oxidized in a process called oxidative phosphorylation.

Conversion of Carbohydrates into Fatty Acids and Cholesterol

The pyruvate produced by glycolysis is an important intermediary in the conversion of carbohydrates into fatty acids and cholesterol. This occurs via the conversion of pyruvate into acetyl-CoA in the mitochondrion. However, this acetyl CoA needs to be transported into cytosol where the synthesis of fatty acids and cholesterol occurs. This cannot occur directly. To obtain cytosolic acetyl-CoA, citrate (produced by the condensation of acetyl CoA with oxaloacetate) is removed from the citric acid cycle and carried across the inner mitochondrial membrane into the cytosol. There it is cleaved by ATP citrate lyase into acetyl-CoA and oxaloacetate. The oxaloacetate is returned to mitochondrion as malate (and then back into oxaloacetate to transfer more acetyl-CoA out of the mitochondrion). The cytosolic acetyl-CoA can be carboxylated by acetyl-CoA carboxylase into malonyl CoA, the first committed step in the synthesis of fatty acids, or it can be combined with acetoacetyl-CoA to form 3-hydroxy-3-methylglutaryl-CoA (HMG-CoA) which is the rate limiting step controlling the synthesis of cholesterol. Cholesterol can be used as is, as a structural component of cellular membranes, or it can be used to synthesize the steroid hormones, bile salts, and vitamin D.

Conversion of Pyruvate into Oxaloacetate for the Citric Acid Cycle

Pyruvate molecules produced by glycolysis are actively transported across the inner mitochondrial membrane, and into the matrix where they can either be oxidized and combined with coenzyme A to form CO_2, acetyl-CoA, and NADH, or they can be carboxylated (by pyruvate carboxylase) to form oxaloacetate. This latter reaction "fills up" the amount of oxaloacetate in the citric acid cycle, and is therefore an anaplerotic reaction (from the Greek meaning to "fill up"), increasing the cycle's capacity to metabolize acetyl-CoA when the tissue's energy needs (e.g. in heart and skeletal muscle) are suddenly increased by activity. In the citric acid cycle all the intermediates (e.g. citrate, iso-citrate, alpha-ketoglutarate, succinate, fumarate, malate and oxaloacetate) are regenerated during each turn of the cycle. Adding more of any of these intermediates to the mitochondrion therefore means that that additional amount is retained within the cycle, increasing all the other intermediates as one is converted into the other. Hence the addition of oxaloacetate greatly increases the amounts of all the citric acid intermediates, thereby increasing the cycle's capacity to metabolize acetyl CoA, converting its acetate component into CO_2 and water, with the release of enough energy to form 11 ATP and 1 GTP molecule for each additional molecule of acetyl CoA that combines with oxaloacetate in the cycle.

To cataplerotically remove oxaloacetate from the citric cycle, malate can be transported from the mitochondrion into the cytoplasm, decreasing the amount of oxaloacetate that can be regenerated. Furthermore, citric acid intermediates are constantly used to form a variety of substances such as the purines, pyrimidines and porphyrins.

Intermediates for Other Pathways

This topic concentrates on the catabolic role of glycolysis with regard to converting potential chemical energy to usable chemical energy during the oxidation of glucose to pyruvate. Many of the metabolites in the glycolytic pathway are also used by anabolic pathways, and, as a consequence, flux through the pathway is critical to maintain a supply of carbon skeletons for biosynthesis.

The following metabolic pathways are all strongly reliant on glycolysis as a source of metabolites:

- Pentose phosphate pathway, which begins with the dehydrogenation of glucose-6-phosphate, the first intermediate to be produced by glycolysis, produces various pentose sugars, and NADPH for the synthesis of fatty acids and cholesterol.
- Glycogen synthesis also starts with glucose-6-phosphate at the beginning of the glycolytic pathway.
- Glycerol, for the formation of triglycerides and phospholipids, is produced from the glycolytic intermediate glyceraldehyde-3-phosphate.
- Various post-glycolytic pathways:
    - Fatty acid synthesis.
    - Cholesterol synthesis.
- The citric acid cycle which in turn leads to:
    - Amino acid synthesis.
    - Nucleotide synthesis.
    - Tetrapyrrole synthesis.

Although gluconeogenesis and glycolysis share many intermediates the one is not functionally a branch or tributary of the other. There are two regulatory steps in both pathways which, when active in the one pathway, are automatically inactive in the other. The two processes can therefore not be simultaneously active. Indeed, if both sets of reactions were highly active at the same time the net result would be the hydrolysis of four high energy phosphate bonds (two ATP and two GTP) per reaction cycle.

NAD^+ is the oxidizing agent in glycolysis, as it is in most other energy yielding metabolic reactions (e.g. beta-oxidation of fatty acids, and during the citric acid cycle). The NADH thus produced is primarily used to ultimately transfer electrons to O_2 to produce water, or, when O_2 is not available, to produced compounds such as lactate or ethanol. NADH is rarely used for synthetic processes, the notable exception being gluconeogenesis. During fatty acid and cholesterol synthesis the reducing agent is NADPH. This difference exemplifies a general principle that NADPH is consumed during biosynthetic reactions, whereas NADH is generated in energy-yielding reactions. The source of the NADPH is two-fold. When malate is oxidatively decarboxylated by "$NADP^+$-linked malic enzyme" pyruvate, CO_2 and NADPH are formed. NADPH is also formed by the pentose phosphate pathway which converts glucose into ribose, which can be used in synthesis of nucleotides and nucleic acids, or it can be catabolized to pyruvate.

Oxidative Phosphorylation

Oxidative phosphorylation is the metabolic pathway in which cells use enzymes to oxidize nutrients, thereby releasing energy which is used to produce adenosine triphosphate (ATP). In most eukaryotes, this takes place inside mitochondria. Almost all aerobic organisms carry out oxidative phosphorylation. This pathway is probably so pervasive because it is a highly efficient way of releasing energy, compared to alternative fermentation processes such as anaerobic glycolysis.

During oxidative phosphorylation, electrons are transferred from electron donors to electron acceptors such as oxygen, in redox reactions. These redox reactions release energy, which is used to form ATP. In eukaryotes, these redox reactions are carried out by a series of protein complexes within the inner membrane of the cell's mitochondria, whereas, in prokaryotes, these proteins are located in the cells' intermembrane space. These linked sets of proteins are called electron transport chains. In eukaryotes, five main protein complexes are involved, whereas in prokaryotes many different enzymes are present, using a variety of electron donors and acceptors.

The energy released by electrons flowing through this electron transport chain is used to transport protons across the inner mitochondrial membrane, in a process called *electron transport*. This generates potential energy in the form of a pH gradient and an electrical potential across this membrane. This store of energy is tapped when protons flow back across the membrane and down the potential energy gradient, through a large enzyme called ATP synthase; this process is known as chemiosmosis. The ATP synthase uses the energy to transform adenosine diphosphate (ADP) into adenosine triphosphate, in a phosphorylation reaction. The reaction is driven by the proton flow, which forces the rotation of a part of the enzyme; the ATP synthase is a rotary mechanical motor.

Although oxidative phosphorylation is a vital part of metabolism, it produces reactive oxygen species such as superoxide and hydrogen peroxide, which lead to propagation of free radicals, damaging cells and contributing to disease and, possibly, aging (senescence). The enzymes carrying out this metabolic pathway are also the target of many drugs and poisons that inhibit their activities.

It is the terminal process of cellular respiration in eukaryotes and accounts for high ATP yield.

Chemiosmosis

Oxidative phosphorylation works by using energy-releasing chemical reactions to drive energy-requiring reactions. The two sets of reactions are said to be *coupled*. This means one cannot occur without the other. The flow of electrons through the electron transport chain, from electron donors such as NADH to electron acceptors such as oxygen, is an exergonic process – it releases energy, whereas the synthesis of ATP is an endergonic process, which requires an input of energy. Both the electron transport chain and the ATP synthase are embedded in a membrane, and energy is transferred from electron transport chain to the ATP synthase by movements of protons across this membrane, in a process called *chemiosmosis*. In practice, this is like a simple electric circuit, with a current of protons being driven from the negative N-side of the membrane to the positive P-side by the proton-pumping enzymes of the electron transport chain. These enzymes are like a battery, as they perform work to drive current through the circuit. The movement of protons creates an electrochemical gradient across the membrane, which is often called the *proton-motive force*. It has two components: a difference in proton concentration (a H^+ gradient, ΔpH) and a difference in electric potential, with the N-side having a negative charge.

ATP synthase releases this stored energy by completing the circuit and allowing protons to flow down the electrochemical gradient, back to the N-side of the membrane. The electrochemical gradient drives the rotation of part of the enzyme's structure and couples this motion to the synthesis of ATP.

The two components of the proton-motive force are thermodynamically equivalent: In mitochondria, the largest part of energy is provided by the potential; in alkaliphile bacteria the electrical energy even has to compensate for a counteracting inverse pH difference. Inversely, chloroplasts operate mainly on ΔpH. However, they also require a small membrane potential for the kinetics of ATP synthesis. In the case of the fusobacterium *Propionigenium modestum* it drives the counter-rotation of subunits a and c of the F_O motor of ATP synthase.

The amount of energy released by oxidative phosphorylation is high, compared with the amount produced by anaerobic fermentation. Glycolysis produces only 2 ATP molecules, but somewhere between 30 and 36 ATPs are produced by the oxidative phosphorylation of the 10 NADH and 2 succinate molecules made by converting one molecule of glucose to carbon dioxide and water, while each cycle of beta oxidation of a fatty acid yields about 14 ATPs. These ATP yields are theoretical maximum values; in practice, some protons leak across the membrane, lowering the yield of ATP.

Electron and Proton Transfer Molecules

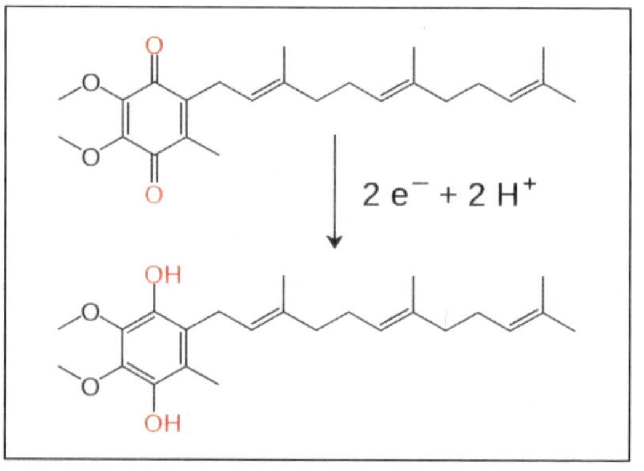

Reduction of coenzyme Q from its ubiquinone form (Q) to the reduced ubiquinol form (QH_2).

The electron transport chain carries both protons and electrons, passing electrons from donors to acceptors, and transporting protons across a membrane. These processes use both soluble and protein-bound transfer molecules. In mitochondria, electrons are transferred within the intermembrane space by the water-soluble electron transfer protein cytochrome c. This carries only electrons, and these are transferred by the reduction and oxidation of an iron atom that the protein holds within a heme group in its structure. Cytochrome c is also found in some bacteria, where it is located within the periplasmic space.

Within the inner mitochondrial membrane, the lipid-soluble electron carrier coenzyme Q10 (Q) carries both electrons and protons by a redox cycle. This small benzoquinone molecule is very hydrophobic, so it diffuses freely within the membrane. When Q accepts two electrons and two protons, it becomes reduced to the *ubiquinol* form (QH_2); when QH_2 releases two electrons and two protons, it becomes oxidized back to the *ubiquinone* (Q) form. As a result, if two enzymes are arranged so that Q is reduced on one side of the membrane and QH_2 oxidized on the other, ubiquinone will couple these reactions and shuttle protons across the membrane. Some bacterial electron transport chains use different quinones, such as menaquinone, in addition to ubiquinone.

Within proteins, electrons are transferred between flavin cofactors, iron–sulfur clusters, and cytochromes. There are several types of iron–sulfur cluster. The simplest kind found in the electron transfer chain consists of two iron atoms joined by two atoms of inorganic sulfur; these are called [2Fe–2S] clusters. The second kind, called [4Fe–4S], contains a cube of four iron atoms and four sulfur atoms. Each iron atom in these clusters is coordinated by an additional amino acid, usually by the sulfur atom of cysteine. Metal ion cofactors undergo redox reactions without binding or releasing protons, so in the electron transport chain they serve solely to transport electrons through proteins. Electrons move quite long distances through proteins by hopping along chains of these cofactors. This occurs by quantum tunnelling, which is rapid over distances of less than 1.4×10^{-9} m.

Eukaryotic Electron Transport Chains

Many catabolic biochemical processes, such as glycolysis, the citric acid cycle, and beta oxidation, produce the reduced coenzyme NADH. This coenzyme contains electrons that have a high transfer potential; in other words, they will release a large amount of energy upon oxidation. However, the cell does not release this energy all at once, as this would be an uncontrollable reaction. Instead, the electrons are removed from NADH and passed to oxygen through a series of enzymes that each release a small amount of the energy. This set of enzymes, consisting of complexes I through IV, is called the electron transport chain and is found in the inner membrane of the mitochondrion. Succinate is also oxidized by the electron transport chain, but feeds into the pathway at a different point.

In eukaryotes, the enzymes in this electron transport system use the energy released from the oxidation of NADH to pump protons across the inner membrane of the mitochondrion. This causes protons to build up in the intermembrane space, and generates an electrochemical gradient across the membrane. The energy stored in this potential is then used by ATP synthase to produce ATP. Oxidative phosphorylation in the eukaryotic mitochondrion is the best-understood example of this process. The mitochondrion is present in almost all eukaryotes, with the exception of anaerobic protozoa such as *Trichomonas vaginalis* that instead reduce protons to hydrogen in a remnant mitochondrion called a hydrogenosome.

Typical respiratory enzymes and substrates in eukaryotes.		
Respiratory enzyme	Redox pair	Midpoint potential (Volts)
NADH dehydrogenase	NAD^+ / NADH	−0.32
Succinate dehydrogenase	FMN or FAD / $FMNH_2$ or $FADH_2$	−0.20
Cytochrome bc_1 complex	Coenzyme $Q10_{ox}$ / Coenzyme $Q10_{red}$	+0.06
Cytochrome bc_1 complex	Cytochrome b_{ox} / Cytochrome b_{red}	+0.12
Complex IV	Cytochrome c_{ox} / Cytochrome c_{red}	+0.22
Complex IV	Cytochrome a_{ox} / Cytochrome a_{red}	+0.29
Complex IV	O_2 / HO^-	+0.82
Conditions: pH = 7		

NADH-Coenzyme Q Oxidoreductase (Complex I)

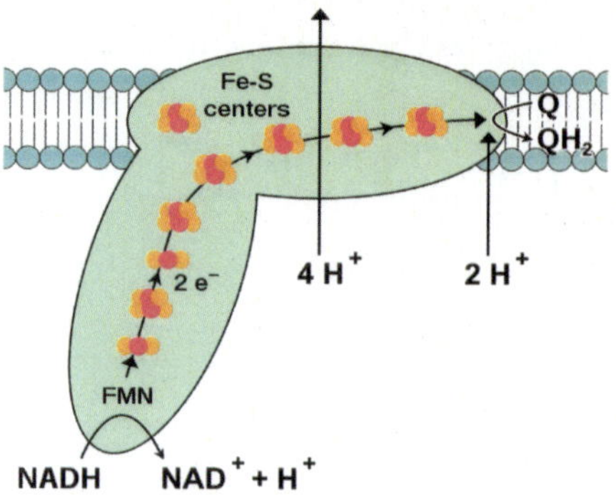

Complex I or NADH-Q oxidoreductase.

NADH-coenzyme Q oxidoreductase, also known as *NADH dehydrogenase* or *complex I*, is the first protein in the electron transport chain. Complex I is a giant enzyme with the mammalian complex I having 46 subunits and a molecular mass of about 1,000 kilodaltons (kDa). The structure is known in detail only from a bacterium; in most organisms the complex resembles a boot with a large "ball" poking out from the membrane into the mitochondrion. The genes that encode the individual proteins are contained in both the cell nucleus and the mitochondrial genome, as is the case for many enzymes present in the mitochondrion.

The reaction that is catalyzed by this enzyme is the two electron oxidation of NADH by coenzyme Q10 or *ubiquinone* (represented as Q in the equation below), a lipid-soluble quinone that is found in the mitochondrion membrane:

$$\mathrm{NADH} + \mathrm{Q} + 5\,\mathrm{H}^{+}{}_{\mathrm{matrix}} \rightarrow \mathrm{NAD}^{+} + \mathrm{QH}_2 + 4\,\mathrm{H}^{+}{}_{\mathrm{intermembrane}}$$

The start of the reaction, and indeed of the entire electron chain, is the binding of a NADH molecule to complex I and the donation of two electrons. The electrons enter complex I via a prosthetic group attached to the complex, flavin mononucleotide (FMN). The addition of electrons to FMN converts it to its reduced form, $FMNH_2$. The electrons are then transferred through a series of iron–sulfur clusters: the second kind of prosthetic group present in the complex. There are both [2Fe–2S] and [4Fe–4S] iron–sulfur clusters in complex I.

As the electrons pass through this complex, four protons are pumped from the matrix into the intermembrane space. Exactly how this occurs is unclear, but it seems to involve conformational changes in complex I that cause the protein to bind protons on the N-side of the membrane and release them on the P-side of the membrane. Finally, the electrons are transferred from the chain of iron–sulfur clusters to a ubiquinone molecule in the membrane. Reduction of ubiquinone also contributes to the generation of a proton gradient, as two protons are taken up from the matrix as it is reduced to ubiquinol (QH_2).

Succinate-Q Oxidoreductase (Complex II)

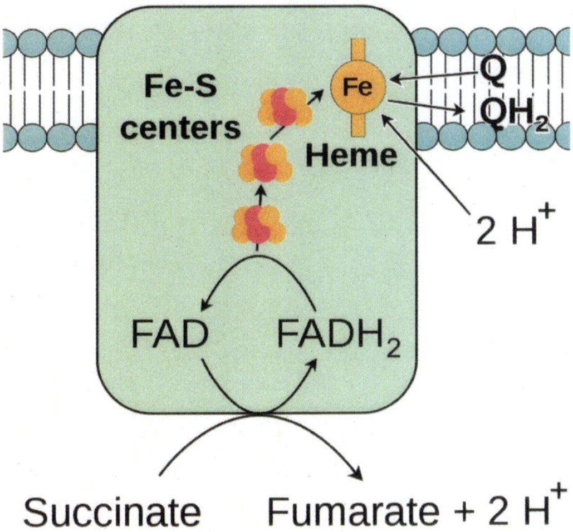

Complex II: Succinate-Q oxidoreductase.

Succinate-Q oxidoreductase, also known as *complex II* or *succinate dehydrogenase*, is a second entry point to the electron transport chain. It is unusual because it is the only enzyme that is part of both the citric acid cycle and the electron transport chain. Complex II consists of four protein subunits and contains a bound flavin adenine dinucleotide (FAD) cofactor, iron–sulfur clusters, and a heme group that does not participate in electron transfer to coenzyme Q, but is believed to be important in decreasing production of reactive oxygen species. It oxidizes succinate to fumarate and reduces ubiquinone. As this reaction releases less energy than the oxidation of NADH, complex II does not transport protons across the membrane and does not contribute to the proton gradient.

$$\text{Succinate} + \text{Q} \rightarrow \text{Fumarate} + \text{QH}_2$$

In some eukaryotes, such as the parasitic worm *Ascaris suum*, an enzyme similar to complex II, fumarate reductase (menaquinol:fumarate oxidoreductase, or QFR), operates in reverse to oxidize ubiquinol and reduce fumarate. This allows the worm to survive in the anaerobic environment of the large intestine, carrying out anaerobic oxidative phosphorylation with fumarate as the electron acceptor. Another unconventional function of complex II is seen in the malaria parasite *Plasmodium falciparum*. Here, the reversed action of complex II as an oxidase is important in regenerating ubiquinol, which the parasite uses in an unusual form of pyrimidine biosynthesis.

Electron Transfer Flavoprotein-Q Oxidoreductase

Electron transfer flavoprotein-ubiquinone oxidoreductase (ETF-Q oxidoreductase), also known as *electron transferring-flavoprotein dehydrogenase*, is a third entry point to the electron transport chain. It is an enzyme that accepts electrons from electron-transferring flavoprotein in the mitochondrial matrix, and uses these electrons to reduce ubiquinone. This enzyme contains a flavin and a [4Fe–4S] cluster, but, unlike the other respiratory complexes, it attaches to the surface of the membrane and does not cross the lipid bilayer.

$$ETF_{red} + Q \rightarrow ETF_{ox} + QH_2$$

In mammals, this metabolic pathway is important in beta oxidation of fatty acids and catabolism of amino acids and choline, as it accepts electrons from multiple acetyl-CoA dehydrogenases. In plants, ETF-Q oxidoreductase is also important in the metabolic responses that allow survival in extended periods of darkness.

Q-Cytochrome C Oxidoreductase (Complex III)

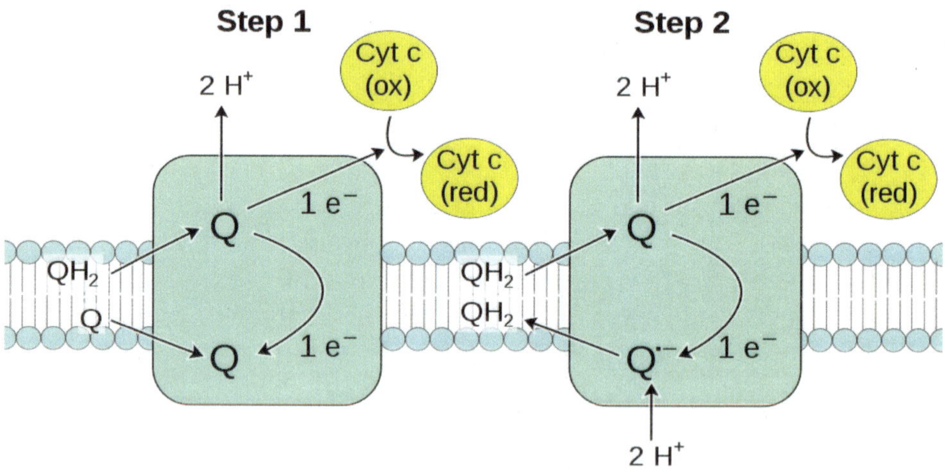

The two electron transfer steps in complex III: Q-cytochrome c oxidoreductase. After each step, Q (in the upper part of the figure) leaves the enzyme.

Q-cytochrome c oxidoreductase is also known as *cytochrome c reductase*, *cytochrome* bc_1 *complex*, or simply *complex III*. In mammals, this enzyme is a dimer, with each subunit complex containing 11 protein subunits, an [2Fe-2S] iron–sulfur cluster and three cytochromes: one cytochrome c_1 and two b cytochromes. A cytochrome is a kind of electron-transferring protein that contains at least one heme group. The iron atoms inside complex III's heme groups alternate between a reduced ferrous (+2) and oxidized ferric (+3) state as the electrons are transferred through the protein.

The reaction catalyzed by complex III is the oxidation of one molecule of ubiquinol and the reduction of two molecules of cytochrome c, a heme protein loosely associated with the mitochondrion. Unlike coenzyme Q, which carries two electrons, cytochrome c carries only one electron.

$$QH_2 + 2\,Cyt\ c_{ox} + 2\,H^+_{matrix} \rightarrow Q + 2\,Cyt\ c_{red} + 4\,H^+_{intermembrane}$$

As only one of the electrons can be transferred from the QH_2 donor to a cytochrome c acceptor at a time, the reaction mechanism of complex III is more elaborate than those of the other respiratory complexes, and occurs in two steps called the Q cycle. In the first step, the enzyme binds three substrates, first, QH_2, which is then oxidized, with one electron being passed to the second substrate, cytochrome c. The two protons released from QH_2 pass into the intermembrane space. The third substrate is Q, which accepts the second electron from the QH_2 and is reduced to $Q^{\cdot -}$, which is the ubisemiquinone free radical. The first two substrates are released, but this ubisemiquinone intermediate remains bound. In the second step, a second molecule of QH_2 is bound and again passes its first electron to a cytochrome c acceptor. The second electron is passed to the bound ubisemiquinone, reducing it to QH_2 as it gains two protons from the mitochondrial matrix. This QH_2 is then released from the enzyme.

As coenzyme Q is reduced to ubiquinol on the inner side of the membrane and oxidized to ubiquinone on the other, a net transfer of protons across the membrane occurs, adding to the proton gradient. The rather complex two-step mechanism by which this occurs is important, as it increases the efficiency of proton transfer. If, instead of the Q cycle, one molecule of QH_2 were used to directly reduce two molecules of cytochrome c, the efficiency would be halved, with only one proton transferred per cytochrome c reduced.

Cytochrome C Oxidase (Complex IV)

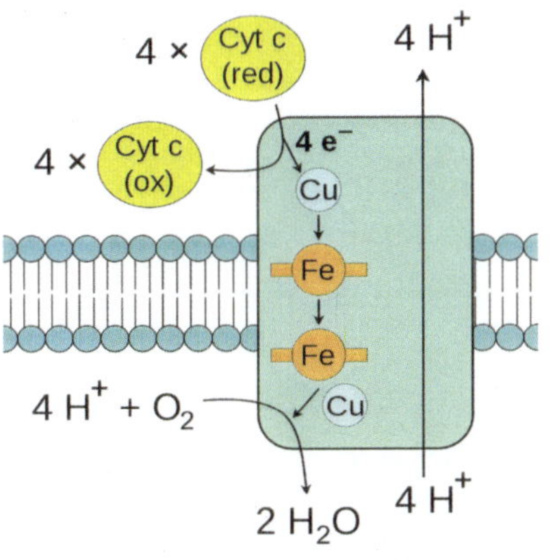

Complex IV: cytochrome c oxidase.

Cytochrome c oxidase, also known as *complex IV*, is the final protein complex in the electron transport chain. The mammalian enzyme has an extremely complicated structure and contains 13 subunits, two heme groups, as well as multiple metal ion cofactors – in all, three atoms of copper, one of magnesium and one of zinc.

This enzyme mediates the final reaction in the electron transport chain and transfers electrons to oxygen, while pumping protons across the membrane. The final electron acceptor oxygen, which is also called the *terminal electron acceptor*, is reduced to water in this step. Both the direct pumping of protons and the consumption of matrix protons in the reduction of oxygen contribute to the proton gradient. The reaction catalyzed is the oxidation of cytochrome c and the reduction of oxygen:

$$4\,\text{Cyt c}_{\text{red}} + O_2 + 8\,H^+_{\text{matrix}} \rightarrow 4\,\text{Cyt c}_{\text{ox}} + 2\,H_2O + 4\,H^+_{\text{intermembrane}}$$

Alternative Reductases and Oxidases

Many eukaryotic organisms have electron transport chains that differ from the much-studied mammalian enzymes described above. For example, plants have alternative NADH oxidases, which oxidize NADH in the cytosol rather than in the mitochondrial matrix, and pass these electrons to the ubiquinone pool. These enzymes do not transport protons, and, therefore, reduce ubiquinone without altering the electrochemical gradient across the inner membrane.

Another example of a divergent electron transport chain is the *alternative oxidase*, which is found in plants, as well as some fungi, protists, and possibly some animals. This enzyme transfers electrons directly from ubiquinol to oxygen.

The electron transport pathways produced by these alternative NADH and ubiquinone oxidases have lower ATP yields than the full pathway. The advantages produced by a shortened pathway are not entirely clear. However, the alternative oxidase is produced in response to stresses such as cold, reactive oxygen species, and infection by pathogens, as well as other factors that inhibit the full electron transport chain. Alternative pathways might, therefore, enhance an organisms' resistance to injury, by reducing oxidative stress.

Organization of Complexes

The original model for how the respiratory chain complexes are organized was that they diffuse freely and independently in the mitochondrial membrane. However, recent data suggest that the complexes might form higher-order structures called supercomplexes or "respirasomes". In this model, the various complexes exist as organized sets of interacting enzymes. These associations might allow channeling of substrates between the various enzyme complexes, increasing the rate and efficiency of electron transfer. Within such mammalian supercomplexes, some components would be present in higher amounts than others, with some data suggesting a ratio between complexes I/II/III/IV and the ATP synthase of approximately 1:1:3:7:4. However, the debate over this supercomplex hypothesis is not completely resolved, as some data do not appear to fit with this model.

Prokaryotic Electron Transport Chains

In contrast to the general similarity in structure and function of the electron transport chains in eukaryotes, bacteria and archaea possess a large variety of electron-transfer enzymes. These use an equally wide set of chemicals as substrates. In common with eukaryotes, prokaryotic electron transport uses the energy released from the oxidation of a substrate to pump ions across a membrane and generate an electrochemical gradient. In the bacteria, oxidative phosphorylation in *Escherichia coli* is understood in most detail, while archaeal systems are at present poorly understood.

The main difference between eukaryotic and prokaryotic oxidative phosphorylation is that bacteria and archaea use many different substances to donate or accept electrons. This allows prokaryotes to grow under a wide variety of environmental conditions. In *E. coli*, for example, oxidative phosphorylation can be driven by a large number of pairs of reducing agents and oxidizing agents, which are listed below. The midpoint potential of a chemical measures how much energy is released when it is oxidized or reduced, with reducing agents having negative potentials and oxidizing agents positive potentials.

Respiratory enzymes and substrates in E. coli.

Respiratory enzyme	Redox pair	Midpoint potential (Volts)
Formate dehydrogenase	Bicarbonate / Formate	−0.43
Hydrogenase	Proton / Hydrogen	−0.42
NADH dehydrogenase	NAD^+ / NADH	−0.32
Glycerol-3-phosphate dehydrogenase	DHAP / Gly-3-P	−0.19
Pyruvate oxidase	Acetate + Carbon dioxide/Pyruvate	?
Lactate dehydrogenase	Pyruvate / Lactate	−0.19
D-amino acid dehydrogenase	2-oxoacid + ammonia/D-amino acid	?
Glucose dehydrogenase	Gluconate/Glucose	−0.14
Succinate dehydrogenase	Fumarate/Succinate	+0.03
Ubiquinol oxidase	Oxygen/Water	+0.82
Nitrate reductase	Nitrate/Nitrite	+0.42
Nitrite reductase	Nitrite/Ammonia	+0.36
Dimethyl sulfoxide reductase	DMSO/DMS	+0.16
Trimethylamine N-oxide reductase	TMAO/TMA	+0.13
Fumarate reductase	Fumarate/ Succinate	+0.03

E. coli can grow with reducing agents such as formate, hydrogen, or lactate as electron donors, and nitrate, DMSO, or oxygen as acceptors. The larger the difference in midpoint potential between an oxidizing and reducing agent, the more energy is released when they react. Out of these compounds, the succinate/fumarate pair is unusual, as its midpoint potential is close to zero. Succinate can therefore be oxidized to fumarate if a strong oxidizing agent such as oxygen is available, or fumarate can be reduced to succinate using a strong reducing agent such as formate. These alternative reactions are catalyzed by succinate dehydrogenase and fumarate reductase, respectively.

Some prokaryotes use redox pairs that have only a small difference in midpoint potential. For example, nitrifying bacteria such as *Nitrobacter* oxidize nitrite to nitrate, donating the electrons to oxygen. The small amount of energy released in this reaction is enough to pump protons and generate ATP, but not enough to produce NADH or NADPH directly for use in anabolism. This problem is solved by using a nitrite oxidoreductase to produce enough proton-motive force to run part of the electron transport chain in reverse, causing complex I to generate NADH.

Prokaryotes control their use of these electron donors and acceptors by varying which enzymes are produced, in response to environmental conditions. This flexibility is possible because different oxidases and reductases use the same ubiquinone pool. This allows many combinations of enzymes to function together, linked by the common ubiquinol intermediate. These respiratory chains therefore have a modular design, with easily interchangeable sets of enzyme systems.

In addition to this metabolic diversity, prokaryotes also possess a range of isozymes – different enzymes that catalyze the same reaction. For example, in *E. coli*, there are two different types of ubiquinol oxidase using oxygen as an electron acceptor. Under highly aerobic conditions, the cell uses an oxidase with a low affinity for oxygen that can transport two protons per electron. However, if levels of oxygen fall, they switch to an oxidase that transfers only one proton per electron, but has a high affinity for oxygen.

ATP Synthase (Complex V)

ATP synthase, also called *complex V*, is the final enzyme in the oxidative phosphorylation pathway. This enzyme is found in all forms of life and functions in the same way in both prokaryotes and eukaryotes. The enzyme uses the energy stored in a proton gradient across a membrane to drive the synthesis of ATP from ADP and phosphate (P_i). Estimates of the number of protons required to synthesize one ATP have ranged from three to four, with some suggesting cells can vary this ratio, to suit different conditions.

$$ADP + P_i + 4\,H^+_{\text{intermembrane}} \rightleftharpoons ATP + H_2O + 4\,H^+_{\text{matrix}}$$

This phosphorylation reaction is an equilibrium, which can be shifted by altering the proton-motive force. In the absence of a proton-motive force, the ATP synthase reaction will run from right to left, hydrolyzing ATP and pumping protons out of the matrix across the membrane. However, when the proton-motive force is high, the reaction is forced to run in the opposite direction; it proceeds from left to right, allowing protons to flow down their concentration gradient and turning ADP into ATP. Indeed, in the closely related vacuolar type H+-ATPases, the hydrolysis reaction is used to acidify cellular compartments, by pumping protons and hydrolysing ATP.

ATP synthase is a massive protein complex with a mushroom-like shape. The mammalian enzyme complex contains 16 subunits and has a mass of approximately 600 kilodaltons. The portion embedded within the membrane is called F_O and contains a ring of c subunits and the proton channel. The stalk and the ball-shaped headpiece is called F_1 and is the site of ATP synthesis. The ball-shaped complex at the end of the F_1 portion contains six proteins of two different kinds (three α subunits and three β subunits), whereas the "stalk" consists of one protein: the γ subunit, with the tip of the stalk extending into the ball of α and β subunits. Both the α and β subunits bind nucleotides, but only the β subunits catalyze the ATP synthesis reaction. Reaching along the side of the F_1 portion and back into the membrane is a long rod-like subunit that anchors the α and β subunits into the base of the enzyme.

As protons cross the membrane through the channel in the base of ATP synthase, the F_0 proton-driven motor rotates. Rotation might be caused by changes in the ionization of amino acids in the ring of c subunits causing electrostatic interactions that propel the ring of c subunits past the proton channel. This rotating ring in turn drives the rotation of the central axle (the γ subunit stalk) within the α and β subunits. The α and β subunits are prevented from rotating themselves by the side-arm, which acts as a stator. This movement of the tip of the γ subunit within the ball of α and β subunits provides the energy for the active sites in the β subunits to undergo a cycle of movements that produces and then releases ATP.

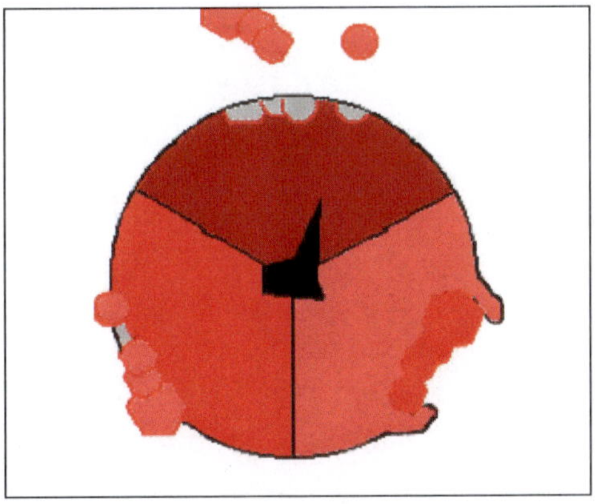

Mechanism of ATP synthase. ATP is shown in red, ADP and phosphate in pink and the rotating γ subunit in black.

This ATP synthesis reaction is called the *binding change mechanism* and involves the active site of a β subunit cycling between three states. In the "open" state, ADP and phosphate enter the active site (shown in brown in the diagram). The protein then closes up around the molecules and binds them loosely – the "loose" state (shown in red). The enzyme then changes shape again and forces these molecules together, with the active site in the resulting "tight" state (shown in pink) binding the newly produced ATP molecule with very high affinity. Finally, the active site cycles back to the open state, releasing ATP and binding more ADP and phosphate, ready for the next cycle.

In some bacteria and archaea, ATP synthesis is driven by the movement of sodium ions through the cell membrane, rather than the movement of protons. Archaea such as *Methanococcus* also contain the A_1A_0 synthase, a form of the enzyme that contains additional proteins with little similarity in sequence to other bacterial and eukaryotic ATP synthase subunits. It is possible that, in some species, the A_1A_0 form of the enzyme is a specialized sodium-driven ATP synthase, but this might not be true in all cases.

Oxidative Phosphorylation- Energetics

The transport of electrons from redox pair NAD^+/ NADH to the final redox pair 1/2 O_2/ H_2O can be summarized as:

$$1/2\ O_2 + NADH + H^+ \rightarrow H_2O + NAD^+$$

The potential difference between this two redox pair is 1.14 Volt which is equivalent to 52 Cal./ Mol.

When one NADH is oxidized through ETC, three ATP are produced which is equal to 21.9 Cal.(7.3 X 3).

The conservation of the energy can be calculated by following formula:

$$\text{Efficiency} = (21.9 \times 100) / 52 = 42\%$$

So we can conclude that when NADH is oxidized, about 42% of energy is conserved in the form of three ATPs and the remaining (58%) energy is lost as heat (entropy).

Reactive Oxygen Species

Molecular oxygen is an ideal terminal electron acceptor because it is a strong oxidizing agent. The reduction of oxygen does involve potentially harmful intermediates. Although the transfer of four electrons and four protons reduces oxygen to water, which is harmless, transfer of one or two electrons produces superoxide or peroxide anions, which are dangerously reactive.

$$O_2 \xrightarrow{e^-} \underset{\text{Superoxide}}{O_2^{\bullet -}} \xrightarrow{e^-} \underset{\text{Peroxide}}{O_2^{2-}}$$

These reactive oxygen species and their reaction products, such as the hydroxyl radical, are very harmful to cells, as they oxidize proteins and cause mutations in DNA. This cellular damage might contribute to disease and is proposed as one cause of aging.

The cytochrome c oxidase complex is highly efficient at reducing oxygen to water, and it releases very few partly reduced intermediates; however small amounts of superoxide anion and peroxide are produced by the electron transport chain. Particularly important is the reduction of coenzyme Q in complex III, as a highly reactive ubisemiquinone free radical is formed as an intermediate in the Q cycle. This unstable species can lead to electron "leakage" when electrons transfer directly to oxygen, forming superoxide.

As the production of reactive oxygen species by these proton-pumping complexes is greatest at high membrane potentials, it has been proposed that mitochondria regulate their activity to maintain the membrane potential within a narrow range that balances ATP production against oxidant generation. For instance, oxidants can activate uncoupling proteins that reduce membrane potential.

To counteract these reactive oxygen species, cells contain numerous antioxidant systems, including antioxidant vitamins such as vitamin C and vitamin E, and antioxidant enzymes such as superoxide dismutase, catalase, and peroxidases, which detoxify the reactive species, limiting damage to the cell.

Inhibitors

There are several well-known drugs and toxins that inhibit oxidative phosphorylation. Although any one of these toxins inhibits only one enzyme in the electron transport chain, inhibition of any step in this process will halt the rest of the process. For example, if oligomycin inhibits ATP synthase, protons cannot pass back into the mitochondrion. As a result, the proton pumps are unable to operate, as the gradient becomes too strong for them to overcome. NADH is then no longer oxidized and the citric acid cycle ceases to operate because the concentration of NAD^+ falls below the concentration that these enzymes can use.

Many site specific inhibitors of ETC have contributed in the present knowledge of the mitochondrial respiration. Synthesis of ATP is also depend on the ETC, so all site specific inhibitors also inhibit ATP formation. Fish poison rotenone, barbitutate drug amytal and antibiotic piercidin A inhibit NADH and coenzyme Q.

Carbon monoxide, cyanide, hydrogen sulphide and azide effectively inhibit cytochrome oxidase. Carbon monoxide reacts with reduced form of the cytochrome while cyanide and azide react with oxidised form. An antibiotic - antimycin A British antile wisite- an antidote used against war-gas re the two important inhibitors of the site between cytochrome B and C1.

Compounds	Use	Site of action	Effect on oxidative phosphorylation
Cyanide Carbon monoxide Azide Hydrogen sulfide	Poisons	Complex IV	Inhibit the electron transport chain by binding more strongly than oxygen to the Fe–Cu center in cytochrome c oxidase, preventing the reduction of oxygen.
Oligomycin	Antibiotic	Complex V	Inhibits ATP synthase by blocking the flow of protons through the F_o subunit.
CCCP 2,4-Dinitrophenol	Poisons, weight-loss	Inner membrane	Ionophores that disrupt the proton gradient by carrying protons across a membrane. This ionophore uncouples proton pumping from ATP synthesis because it carries protons across the inner mitochondrial membrane.

Rotenone	Pesticide	Complex I	Prevents the transfer of electrons from complex I to ubiquinone by blocking the ubiquinone-binding site.
Malonate and oxaloacetate	Poisons	Complex II	Competitive inhibitors of succinate dehydrogenase (complex II).
Antimycin A	Piscicide	Complex III	Binds to the Qi site of cytochrome c reductase, thereby inhibiting the oxidation of ubiquinol.

Not all inhibitors of oxidative phosphorylation are toxins. In brown adipose tissue, regulated proton channels called uncoupling proteins can uncouple respiration from ATP synthesis. This rapid respiration produces heat, and is particularly important as a way of maintaining body temperature for hibernating animals, although these proteins may also have a more general function in cells' responses to stress.

Citric Acid Cycle

The citric acid cycle (also known as the Krebs Cycle) is actually a part of the much larger process called cellular respiration, the process where your body harvests energy from the food you eat. Yes, the citric acid cycle has the same citric acid found in oranges and other citrus fruits.

Where does the citric acid cycle fit into cellular respiration?

1. Glycolysis, where the simple sugar glucose is broken down, occurs in the cytosol.
2. Pyruvate, the product from glycolysis, is transformed into acetyl CoA in the mitochondria for the next step.
3. The citric acid cycle, where acetyl CoA is modified in the mitochondria to produce energy precursors in preparation for the next step.
4. Oxidative phosphorylation, the process where electron transport from the energy precursors from the citric acid cycle (step 3) leads to the phosphorylation of ADP, producing ATP. This also occurs in the mitochondria.

The citric acid cycle captures the energy stored in the chemical bonds of acetyl. CoA (processed glucose) in a step-by-step process, trapping it in the form of high-energy intermediate molecules. The trapped energy from the citric acid cycle is then passed on to oxidative phosphorylation, where it is converted to a usable form of cellular energy, ATP (adenosine triphosphate). We can then use that energy to move, breathe, make our hearts beat, and think (among other things).

How does it Happen?

The molecules that enter and circulate through the citric acid cycle are made mostly of carbon atoms. To understand how the citric acid cycle works, we need to follow how the carbon atoms are rearranged through the cycle. Molecules, called electron shuttles, accept the energy released by stepwise rearrangements and the subtraction of carbons in the form of electrons. Electron shuttles are small organic molecules, such as $NAD^+$and FADH, that transport high energy electrons to where they need to be by gaining electrons (through "reduction") and losing electrons (through "oxidation"). The electrons transported by electron shuttles will later be used to generate ATP.

Some of the Key Players in the Citric Acid Cycle are:

Energy Shuttles

1. NADH: An energy shuttle which delivers high energy electrons to the electron transport chain where they will eventually power the production of 2 to 3 ATP molecules. When this electron shuttle is not carrying high energy electrons, meaning it has been oxidized (lost its electrons), it is left with a positive charge and is called NAD^+.

2. $FADH_2$: Another energy shuttle that carries high energy electrons to the electron transport chain, where they will ultimately drive production of 1 to 2 ATP molecules. The oxidized form of $FADH_2$ is FAD and happens just like in NADH.

High Energy Molecules

1. ATP: The basic energy currency of the cell. It's a form of energy that cells can use right away.

2. GTP: Similar to ATP, GTP can be easily converted to ATP in the cell.

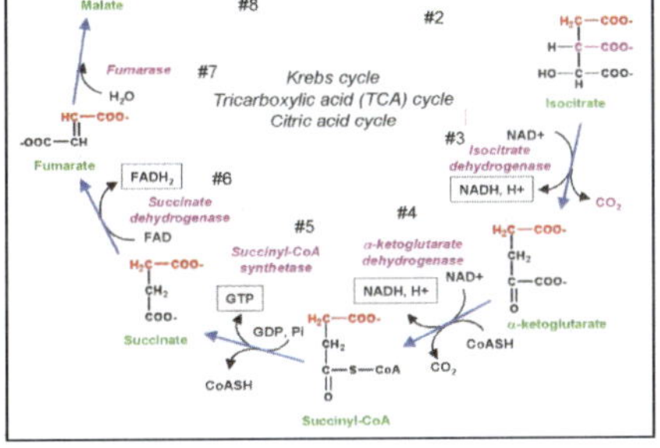

Step 1: Glycolysis - A 6-carbon glucose molecule is split into two 3-carbon molecules called pyruvates. Pyruvate is needed in order to create acetyl CoA.

Step 2: The transformation of pyruvate to acetyl CoA - This is a very short step in between glycolysis and the citric acid cycle. The 3-carbon pyruvate molecule made in glycolysis loses a carbon to produce a new, 2-carbon molecule called acetyl CoA. The carbon that is removed takes two oxygens from pyruvate with it, and exits the body as carbon dioxide (CO_2. CO_2, end subscript is the waste product that you release when you exhale.

Step 3: The citric acid cycle - The citric acid cycle is called a cycle because the starting molecule, oxaloacetate (which has 4 carbons), is regenerated at the end of the cycle. Throughout the citric acid cycle, oxaloacetate is progressively transformed into several different molecules (as carbon atoms are added to and removed from it), but at the end of the cycle it always turns back into oxaloacetate to be used again. Energy can be captured from this cycle because several of the steps are energetically favourable. When a step is favoured, it means that the products of the reaction have lower energy than the reactants. The difference in energy between the products and the reactants is the energy that is released when the reaction takes place. The released energy is captured as the electron shuttles (NAD^+ and FAD) are reduced to NADH and $FADH_2$.

To start the cycle, an enzyme fuses acetyl CoA and oxaloacetate together so that citric acid is formed (a 2-carbon molecule + a 4-carbon molecule = a 6-carbon molecule). This is the first molecule that is made in the cycle and is where the cycle gets its name. Enzymes then proceed to speed up (or "catalyze") a sequence of rearrangements that convert the newly made citric acid molecule into a series of slightly different molecules. These enzymes only change the rate that these rearrangements occur, not the outcome:

1. An enzyme rearranges the atoms in the citric acid molecule (6 carbons) into a new 6-carbon arrangement.

2. Energy is released when the 6-carbon arrangement is oxidized, causing one carbon to be removed. The removed carbon molecule combines with oxygen to produce CO_2 Some of the energy, in the form of electrons, is captured in formation of high-energy compound, NADH. (Recall that some of the energy released from the cycle is used to reduce NAD^+ to create NADH.) The high energy electrons that are handed to NAD^+ for reduction come from the oxidation (loss of electrons) from the carbon molecule here.

3. Next, the same type of reaction happens again. Another carbon is cleaved off the 5-carbon molecule, leaving a 4-carbon molecule and CO_2, and some of the energy released is used to reduce NAD^+ to NADH.

4. Rearrangement occurs, allowing the 4-carbon molecule to find a more comfortable configuration (one that doesn't use require a lot of energy or structural strain, and one that allows each bond to be satisfied). During this rearrangement, non-carbon groups are added to and removed from the molecule. GTP and $FADH_2$ are made in these steps.

5. The 4-carbon molecule rearranges its carbons one last time, producing oxaloacetate. Remember that oxaloacetate will be used again in the next cycle. Once again, some of the energy released is transferred to reduce NAD^+ to NADH.

The products of the citric acid cycle: From one citric acid cycle, the following products are formed:

- 1 GTP,
- 3 NADH,
- 1 $FADH_2$,
- 2 CO_2,
- Regenerated oxaloacetate.

The CO_2 that is released during the transformation step (step 2) and the two CO_2 that are made during the citric acid cycle are the same three carbons that came from the initial pyruvate (made at the end of step 1 of cellular respiration). After two rounds of the citric acid cycle, we have completely oxidized one molecule of glucose to CO_2 and captured its energy in a series of steps. These products from the citric acid cycle are made in the mitochondria of your cells.

Step 4: Oxidative phosphorylation - During oxidative phosphorylation, NADH and $FADH_2$ are transported to the electron transport chain, where their high energy electrons will ultimately drive synthesis of ATP.

References

- Goldman, Lee, MD; Schafer, Andrew I., MD (2016). Goldman-Cecil Medicine, Twenty-Fifth Edition. Philadelphia, PA: Elsevier. pp. 1458–1466. ISBN 978-1-4557-5017-7
- Metabolism, science: britannica.com, Retrieved 10 March, 2019
- Maroon, J; Bost J; Amos A; Zuccoli G (May 2013). "Restricted Calorie Ketogenic Diet for the Treatment of Glioblastoma Multiforme". Journal of Child Neurology. 28 (8): 1002–1008. doi:10.1177/0883073813488670. PMID 23670248
- Ragland, S.S.; Sohal, R.S. (1975). "Ambient temperature, physical activity and aging in the housefly, Musca domestica". Experimental Gerontology. 10 (5): 279–89. doi:10.1016/0531-5565(75)90005-4. PMID 1204688

- Atp-important-molecule-in-metabolism-4050962: thoughtco.com, Retrieved 15 June, 2019
- Biomolecules, test-prep, krebs-citric-acid-cycle-and-oxidative-phosphorylation, the-citric-acid-cycle-2: khanacademy.org, Retrieved 26 May, 2019
- Berg, Jeremy M.; Tymoczko, John L.; Stryer, Lubert; Gatto, Gregory J. (2012). Biochemistry (7th ed.). New York: W.H. Freeman. pp. 480–482. ISBN 9781429229364

3

Macronutrients and their Metabolism

Some of the major macronutrients which are present in the body are carbohydrates, fats and proteins. Their metabolism refers to the various biochemical processes due to which the formation, breakdown and interconversion of these macronutrients takes place within living organisms. This chapter discusses in detail the processes related to the metabolism of these macronutrients.

Carbohydrate

Carbohydrates are the sugars, starches and fibers found in fruits, grains, vegetables and milk products. Though often maligned in trendy diets, carbohydrates — one of the basic food groups — are important to a healthy diet.

"Carbohydrates are macronutrients, meaning they are one of the three main ways the body obtains energy, or calories", carbohydrates are the body's main source of energy. They are called carbohydrates because, at the chemical level, they contain carbon, hydrogen and oxygen.

There are three macronutrients: carbohydrates, protein and fats. Macronutrients are essential for proper body functioning, and the body requires large amounts of them. All macronutrients must be obtained through diet; the body cannot produce macronutrients on its own.

The recommended daily amount (RDA) of carbs for adults is 135 grams, however, the NIH also recommends that everyone should have his or her own carbohydrate goal. Carb intake for most people should be between 45% and 65% of total calories. One gram of carbohydrates equals about 4 calories, so a diet of 1,800 calories per day would equal about 202 grams on the low end and 292 grams of carbs on the high end. However, people with diabetes should not eat more than 200 grams of carbs per day, while pregnant women need at least 175 grams.

Functions of Carbohydrates

Carbohydrates provide fuel for the central nervous system and energy for working muscles. They also prevent protein from being used as an energy source and enable fat metabolism.

Also, carbohydrates are important for brain function. They are an influence on "mood, memory, etc., as well as a quick energy source." In fact, the RDA of carbohydrates is based on the amount of carbs the brain needs to function.

Simple vs. Complex Carbohydrates

Carbohydrates are classified as simple or complex. The difference between the two forms is the chemical structure and how quickly the sugar is absorbed and digested. Generally speaking, simple carbs are digested and absorbed more quickly and easily than complex carbs.

Simple carbohydrates contain just one or two sugars, such as fructose (found in fruits) and galactose (found in milk products). These single sugars are called monosaccharides. Carbs with two sugars — such as sucrose (table sugar), lactose (from dairy) and maltose (found in beer and some vegetables) — are called disaccharides.

Simple carbs are also in candy, soda and syrups. However, these foods are made with processed and refined sugars and do not have vitamins, minerals or fiber. They are called "empty calories" and can lead to weight gain.

Complex carbohydrates (polysaccharides) have three or more sugars. They are often referred to as starchy foods and include beans, peas, lentils, peanuts, potatoes, corn, parsnips, whole-grain breads and cereals.

Smathers pointed out that, while all carbohydrates function as relatively quick energy sources, simple carbs cause bursts of energy much more quickly than complex carbs because of the quicker rate at which they are digested and absorbed. Simple carbs can lead to spikes in blood sugar levels and sugar highs, while complex carbs provide more sustained energy.

Studies have shown that replacing saturated fats with simple carbs, such as those in many processed foods, is associated with an increased risk of heart disease and type 2 diabetes.

It's best to focus on getting primarily complex carbs in your diet, including whole grains and vegetables.

Sugars, Starches and Fibers

In the body, carbs break down into smaller units of sugar, such as glucose and fructose. The small intestine absorbs these smaller units, which then enter the bloodstream and travel to the liver. The liver converts all of these sugars into glucose, which is carried through the bloodstream — accompanied by insulin — and converted into energy for basic body functioning and physical activity.

If the glucose is not immediately needed for energy, the body can store up to 2,000 calories of it in the liver and skeletal muscles in the form of glycogen. Once glycogen stores are full, carbs are stored as fat. If you have insufficient carbohydrate intake or stores, the body will consume protein for fuel. This is problematic because the body needs protein to make muscles. Using protein instead of carbohydrates for fuel also puts stress on the kidneys, leading to the passage of painful byproducts in the urine.

Fiber is essential to digestion. Fibers promote healthy bowel movements and decrease the risk of chronic diseases such as coronary heart disease and diabetes. However, unlike sugars and starches, fibers are not absorbed in the small intestine and are not converted to glucose. Instead, they pass into the large intestine relatively intact, where they are converted to hydrogen and carbon dioxide and fatty acids. The Institute of Medicine recommends that people consume 14 grams of fiber for every 1,000 calories. Sources of fiber include fruits, grains and vegetables, especially legumes.

Carbs are also found naturally in some forms of dairy and both starchy and nonstarchy vegetables. For example, nonstarchy vegetables like lettuces, kale, green beans, celery, carrots and broccoli all contain carbs. Starchy vegetables like potatoes and corn also contain carbohydrates, but in larger amounts. nonstarchy vegetables generally contain only about 5 grams of carbohydrates per cup of raw vegetables, and most of those carbs come from fiber.

Good Carbs vs. Bad Carbs

Carbohydrates are found in foods you know are good for you (vegetables) and ones you know are not (doughnuts). This has led to the idea that some carbs are "good" and some are "bad". carbs commonly considered bad include pastries, sodas, highly processed foods, white rice, white bread and other white-flour foods. These are foods with simple carbs. Bad carbs rarely have any nutritional value.

Carbs usually considered good are complex carbs, such as whole grains, fruits, vegetables, beans and legumes. These are not only processed more slowly, but they also contain a bounty of other nutrients.

Good carbs are:

- Low or moderate in calories.
- High in nutrients.
- Devoid of refined sugars and refined grains.

- High in naturally occurring fiber.
- Low in sodium.
- Low in saturated fat.
- Very low in, or devoid of, cholesterol and trans fats.

Bad carbs are:

- High in calories.
- Full of refined sugars, like corn syrup, white sugar, honey and fruit juices.
- High in refined grains like white flour.
- Low in many nutrients.
- Low in fiber.
- High in sodium.
- Sometimes high in saturated fat.
- Sometimes high in cholesterol and trans fats.

Carbohydrate Benefits

The right kind of carbs can be incredibly good for you. Not only are they necessary for your health, but they carry a variety of added benefits.

Mental Health

Carbohydrates may be important to mental health. People on a high-fat, low-carb diet for a year had more anxiety, depression and anger than people on a low-fat, high-carb diet. Scientists suspect that carbohydrates help with the production of serotonin in the brain.

Carbs may help memory, too. The women on no-carb diets did worse than overweight women on low-calorie diets that contained a healthy amount of carbohydrates.

Weight Loss

Though carbs are often blamed for weight gain, the right kind of carbs can actually help you lose and maintain a healthy weight. This happens because many good carbohydrates, especially whole grains and vegetables with skin, contain fiber. It is difficult to get sufficient fiber on a low-carb diet. Dietary fiber helps you to feel full, and generally comes in relatively low-calorie foods.

A study followed middle-age women for 20 months and found that participants who ate more fiber lost weight, while those who decreased their fiber intake gained weight. Another recent study linked fat loss with low-fat diets, not low-carb ones.

While some studies have found that low-carb diets do help people lose weight, a meta analysis conducted in 2015 and published in The Lancet found that when viewed long term, low-fat and low-carb diets had similar success rates. People lost more weight early on while on low-carb diets but after a year they were all in similar places.

Good Source of Nutrients

Whole, unprocessed fruits and vegetables are well known for their nutrient content. Some are even considered superfoods because of it — and all of these leafy greens, bright sweet potatoes, juicy berries, tangy citruses and crunchy apples contain carbs.

One important, plentiful source of good carbs is whole grains. A large study found that those eating the most whole grains had significantly higher amounts of fiber, energy and polyunsaturated fats, as well as all micronutrients (except vitamin B12 and sodium). An additional studyfound that whole grains contain antioxidants, which were previously thought to exist almost exclusively in fruits and vegetables.

Heart Health

Fiber also helps to lower cholesterol. The digestive process requires bile acids, which are made partly with cholesterol. As your digestion improves, the liver pulls cholesterol from the blood to create more bile acid, thereby reducing the amount of LDL, the "bad" cholesterol.

Toups referenced a study that looked at the effect of whole grains on patients taking cholesterol-lowering medications called statins. Those who ate more than 16 grams of whole grains daily had lower bad-cholesterol levels than those who took the statins without eating the whole grains.

Carbohydrate Deficiency

Not getting enough carbs can cause problems. Without sufficient fuel, the body gets no energy. Additionally, without sufficient glucose, the central nervous system suffers, which may cause dizziness or mental and physical weakness. A deficiency of glucose, or low blood sugar, is called hypoglycemia.

If the body has insufficient carbohydrate intake or stores, it will consume protein for fuel. This is problematic because the body needs protein to make muscles. Using protein for fuel instead of carbohydrates also puts stress on the kidneys, leading to the passage of painful byproducts in the urine.

People who don't consume enough carbohydrates may also suffer from insufficient fiber, which can cause digestive problems and constipation.

Carbohydrate Metabolism

Carbohydrate metabolism is the whole of biochemical processes responsible for the metabolic formation, breakdown, and interconversion of carbohydrates in living organisms.

Carbohydrates are central to many essential metabolic pathways. Plants synthesize carbohydrates from carbon dioxide and water through photosynthesis, allowing them to store energy absorbed from sunlight internally. When animals and fungi consume plants, they use cellular respiration to break down these stored carbohydrates to make energy available to cells. Both animals and plants temporarily store the released energy in the form of high energy molecules, such as ATP, for use in various cellular processes.

Although humans consume a variety of carbohydrates, digestion breaks down complex carbohydrates into a few simple monomers (monosaccharides) for metabolism: glucose, fructose, and galactose. Glucose constitutes about 80% of the products, and is the primary structure that is distributed to cells in the tissues, where it is broken down or stored as glycogen. In aerobic respiration, the main form of cellular respiration used by humans, glucose and oxygen are metabolized to release energy, with carbon dioxide and water as byproducts. Most of the fructose and galactose travel to the liver, where they can be converted to glucose.

Some simple carbohydrates have their own enzymatic oxidation pathways, as do only a few of the more complex carbohydrates. The disaccharide lactose, for instance, requires the enzyme lactase to be broken into its monosaccharide components, glucose and galactose.

Metabolic Pathways

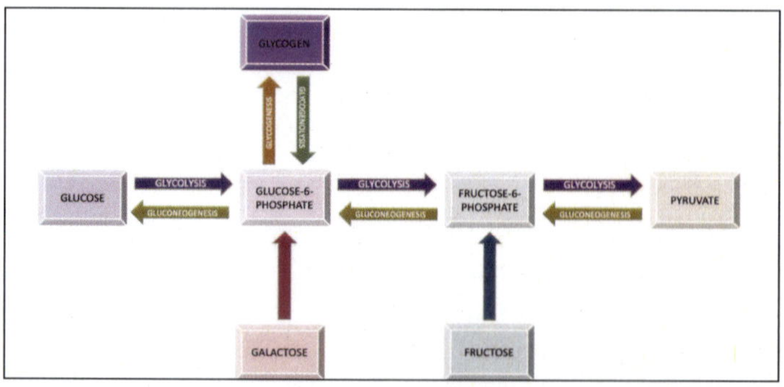

Overview of connections between metabolic processes.

Glycolysis

Glycolysis is the process of breaking down a glucose molecule into two pyruvate molecules, while storing energy released during this process as ATP and NADH. Nearly all organisms that break down glucose utilize glycolysis. Glucose regulation and product use are the primary categories in which these pathways differ between organisms. In some tissues and organisms, glycolysis is the sole method of energy production. This pathway is common to both anaerobic and aerobic respiration.

Glycolysis consists of ten steps, split into two phases. During the first phase, it requires the breakdown of two ATP molecules. During the second phase, chemical energy from the intermediates is transferred into ATP and NADH. The breakdown of one molecule of glucose results in two molecules of pyruvate, which can be further oxidized to access more energy in later processes.

Gluconeogenesis

Gluconeogenesis is the reverse process of glycolysis. It involves the conversion of non-carbohydrate molecules into glucose. The non-carbohydrate molecules that are converted in this pathway include pyruvate, lactate, glycerol, alanine, and glutamine. This process occurs when there are lowered amounts of glucose. The liver is the primary location of gluconeogenesis, but some also occurs in the kidney.

This pathway is regulated by multiple different molecules. Glucagon, adrenocorticotropic hormone, and ATP encourage gluconeogenesis. Gluconeogenesis is inhibited by AMP, ADP, and insulin.

Glycogenolysis

Glycogenolysis refers to the breakdown of glycogen. In the liver, muscles, and the kidney, this process occurs to provide glucose when necessary. A single glucose molecule is cleaved from a branch of glycogen, and is transformed into glucose-1-phosphate during this process. This molecule can then be converted to glucose-6-phosphate, an intermediate in the glycolysis pathway.

Glucose-6-phosphate can then progress through glycolysis. Glycolysis only requires the input of one molecule of ATP when the glucose originates in glycogen. Alternatively, glucose-6-phosphate can be converted back into glucose in the liver and the kidneys, allowing it to raise blood glucose levels if necessary.

Glucagon in the liver stimulates glycogenolysis when the blood glucose is lowered, known as hypoglycemia. The glycogen in the liver can function as a backup source of glucose between meals. Adrenaline stimulates the breakdown of glycogen in the skeletal muscle during exercise. In the muscles, glycogen ensures a rapidly accessible energy source for movement.

Glycogenesis

Glycogenesis refers to the process of synthesizing glycogen. In humans, excess glucose is converted to glycogen via this process. Glycogen is a highly branched structure, consisting of glucose, in the form of glucose-6-phosphate, linked together. The branching of glycogen increases its solubility, and allows for a higher number of glucose molecules to be accessible for breakdown. Glycogenesis occurs primarily in the liver, skeletal muscles, and kidney.

Pentose Phosphate Pathway

The pentose phosphate pathway is an alternative method of oxidizing glucose. It occurs in the liver, adipose tissue, adrenal cortex, testis, milk glands, phagocyte cells, and red blood cells. It produces products that are used in other cell processes, while reducing NADP to NADPH. This pathway is regulated through changes in the activity of glucose-6-phosphate dehydrogenase.

Fructose Metabolism

Fructose must undergo certain extra steps in order to enter the glycolysis pathway. Enzymes located in certain tissues can add a phosphate group to fructose. This phosphorylation creates fructose-6-phosphate, an intermediate in the glycolysis pathway that can be broken down directly in those tissues. This pathway occurs in the muscles, adipose tissue, and kidney. In the liver, enzymes produce fructose-1-phosphate, which enters the glycolysis pathway and is later cleaved into glyceraldehyde and dihydroxyacetone phosphate.

Galactose Metabolism

Lactose, or milk sugar, consists of one molecule of glucose and one molecule of galactose. After separation from glucose, galactose travels to the liver for conversion to glucose. Galactokinase uses one molecule of ATP to phosphorylate galactose. The phosphorylated galactose is then converted to glucose-1-phosphate, and then eventually glucose-6-phosphate, which can be broken down in glycolysis.

Energy Production

Many steps of carbohydrate metabolism allow the cells to access energy, and store it more transiently in ATP. The cofactors NAD^+ and FAD are sometimes reduced during this process to form NADH and $FADH_2$, which drive the creation of ATP in other processes. A molecule of NADH can produce 1.5–2.5 molecules of ATP, whereas a molecule of $FADH_2$ will yield 1.5 molecules of ATP.

Energy produced during metabolism of one glucose molecule						
Pathway	ATP Input	ATP Output	Net ATP	NADH Output	$FADH_2$ Output	ATP Final Yield
Glycolysis (aerobic)	2	4	2	2	0	5-7
Citric Acid Cycle	0	2	2	8	2	17-25

Typically, the complete breakdown of one molecule of glucose via aerobic respiration (i.e. involving both glycolysis and the Citric Acid Cycle) is usually about 30–32 molecules of ATP. Oxidation of one gram of carbohydrate yields approximately 4 kcal of energy.

Hormonal Regulation

Glucoregulation is the maintenance of steady levels of glucose in the body. Hormones released from the pancreas regulate the overall metabolism of glucose. Insulin and glucagon are the primary hormones involved in maintaining a steady level of glucose in the blood, and the release of each is controlled by the amount of nutrients currently available. The amount of insulin released in the blood and sensitivity of the cells to the insulin both determine the amount of glucose that cells break down. Increased levels of glucagon activates the enzymes that catalyze glycogenolysis, and inhibits the enzymes that catalyze glycogenesis. Conversely, glycogenesis is enhanced and glycogenolysis inhibited when there are high levels of insulin in the blood.

The level of circulatory glucose (known informally as "blood sugar") is the most important factor determining the amount of glucagon or insulin produced. The release of glucagon is precipitated by low levels of blood glucose, whereas high levels of blood glucose stimulates cells to produce insulin. Because the level of circulatory glucose is largely determined by the intake of dietary carbohydrates, diet controls major aspects of metabolism via insulin. In humans, insulin is made by beta cells in the pancreas, fat is stored in adipose tissue cells, and glycogen is both stored and released as needed by liver cells. Regardless of insulin levels, no glucose is released to the blood from internal glycogen stores from muscle cells.

Carbohydrates as Storage

Carbohydrates are typically stored as long polymers of glucose molecules with glycosidic bonds for structural support (e.g. chitin, cellulose) or for energy storage (e.g. glycogen, starch). However, the strong affinity of most carbohydrates for water makes storage of large quantities of carbohydrates inefficient due to the large molecular weight of the solvated water-carbohydrate complex. In most organisms, excess carbohydrates are regularly catabolised to form acetyl-CoA, which is a feed stock for the fatty acid synthesis pathway; fatty acids, triglycerides, and other lipids are commonly used for long-term energy storage. The hydrophobic character of lipids makes them a much more compact form of energy storage than hydrophilic carbohydrates. However, animals, including humans, lack the necessary enzymatic machinery and so do not synthesize glucose from lipids (with a few exceptions, e.g. glycerol).

In some animals (such as termites) and some microorganisms (such as protists and bacteria), cellulose can be disassembled during digestion and absorbed as glucose.

Protein

Proteins are large biomolecules, or macromolecules, consisting of one or more long chains of amino acid residues. Proteins perform a vast array of functions within organisms, including catalysing metabolic reactions, DNA replication, responding to stimuli, providing structure to cells and organisms, and transporting molecules from one location to another. Proteins differ from one another primarily in their sequence of amino acids, which is dictated by the nucleotide sequence of their genes, and which usually results in protein folding into a specific three-dimensional structure that determines its activity.

A linear chain of amino acid residues is called a polypeptide. A protein contains at least one long polypeptide. Short polypeptides, containing less than 20–30 residues, are rarely considered to be proteins and are commonly called peptides, or sometimes oligopeptides. The individual amino acid residues are bonded together by peptide bonds and adjacent amino acid residues. The sequence of amino acid residues in a protein is defined by the sequence of a gene, which is encoded in the genetic code. In general, the genetic code specifies 20 standard amino acids; however, in certain organisms the genetic code can include selenocysteine and—in certain archaea—pyrrolysine. Shortly after or even during synthesis, the residues in a protein are often chemically modified by post-translational modification, which alters the physical and chemical properties, folding, stability, activity, and ultimately, the function of the proteins. Sometimes proteins have non-peptide groups attached, which can be called prosthetic groups or cofactors. Proteins can also work together to achieve a particular function, and they often associate to form stable protein complexes.

Once formed, proteins only exist for a certain period and are then degraded and recycled by the cell's machinery through the process of protein turnover. A protein's lifespan is measured in terms of its half-life and covers a wide range. They can exist for minutes or years with an average lifespan of 1–2 days in mammalian cells. Abnormal or misfolded proteins are degraded more rapidly either due to being targeted for destruction or due to being unstable.

Like other biological macromolecules such as polysaccharides and nucleic acids, proteins are essential parts of organisms and participate in virtually every process within cells. Many proteins are enzymes that catalyse biochemical reactions and are vital to metabolism. Proteins also have structural or mechanical functions, such as actin and myosin in muscle and the proteins in the cytoskeleton, which form a system of scaffolding that maintains cell shape. Other proteins are important in cell signaling, immune responses, cell adhesion, and the cell cycle. In animals, proteins are needed in the diet to provide the essential amino acids that cannot be synthesized. Digestion breaks the proteins down for use in the metabolism.

Proteins may be purified from other cellular components using a variety of techniques such as ultracentrifugation, precipitation, electrophoresis, and chromatography; the advent of genetic engineering has made possible a number of methods to facilitate purification. Methods commonly used to study protein structure and function include immunohistochemistry, site-directed mutagenesis, X-ray crystallography, nuclear magnetic resonance and mass spectrometry.

Structure

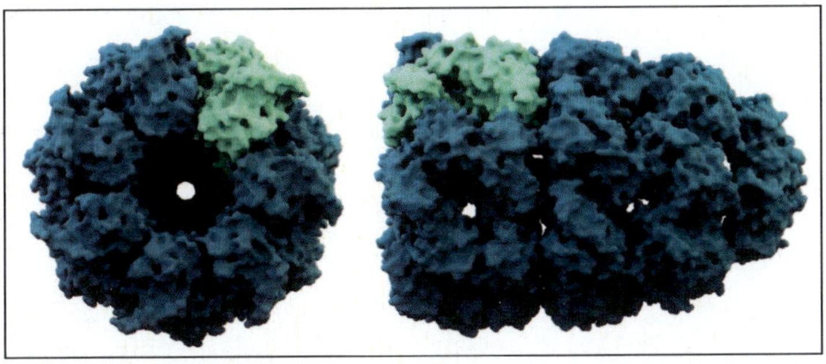

The crystal structure of the chaperonin, a huge protein complex. A single protein subunit is highlighted. Chaperonins assist protein folding.

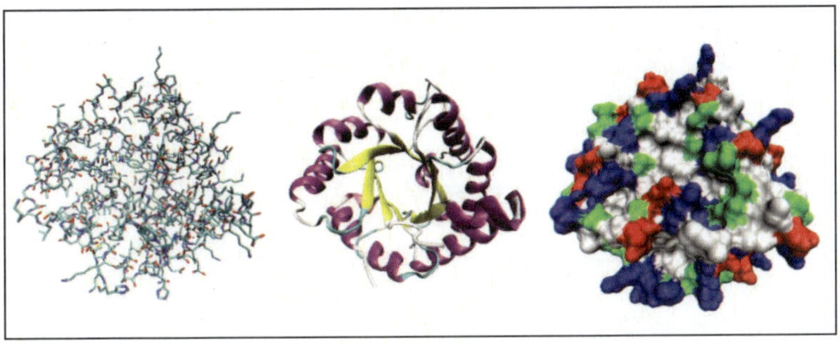

Three possible representations of the three-dimensional structure of the protein triose phosphate isomerase. Left: All-atom representation colored by atom type. Middle: Simplified representation illustrating the backbone conformation, colored by secondary structure. Right: Solvent-accessible surface representation colored by residue type (acidic residues red, basic residues blue, polar residues green, nonpolar residues white).

Most proteins fold into unique 3-dimensional structures. The shape into which a protein naturally folds is known as its native conformation. Although many proteins can fold unassisted, simply through the chemical properties of their amino acids, others require the aid of molecular chaperones to fold into their native states. Biochemists often refer to four distinct aspects of a protein's structure:

- *Primary structure*: the amino acid sequence. A protein is a polyamide.
- *Secondary structure*: regularly repeating local structures stabilized by hydrogen bonds. The most common examples are the α-helix, β-sheet and turns. Because secondary structures are local, many regions of different secondary structure can be present in the same protein molecule.

- *Tertiary structure*: the overall shape of a single protein molecule; the spatial relationship of the secondary structures to one another. Tertiary structure is generally stabilized by nonlocal interactions, most commonly the formation of a hydrophobic core, but also through salt bridges, hydrogen bonds, disulfide bonds, and even posttranslational modifications. The term "tertiary structure" is often used as synonymous with the term *fold*. The tertiary structure is what controls the basic function of the protein.
- *Quaternary structure*: the structure formed by several protein molecules (polypeptide chains), usually called *protein subunits* in this context, which function as a single protein complex.

Proteins are not entirely rigid molecules. In addition to these levels of structure, proteins may shift between several related structures while they perform their functions. In the context of these functional rearrangements, these tertiary or quaternary structures are usually referred to as "conformations", and transitions between them are called *conformational changes*. Such changes are often induced by the binding of a substrate molecule to an enzyme's active site, or the physical region of the protein that participates in chemical catalysis. In solution proteins also undergo variation in structure through thermal vibration and the collision with other molecules.

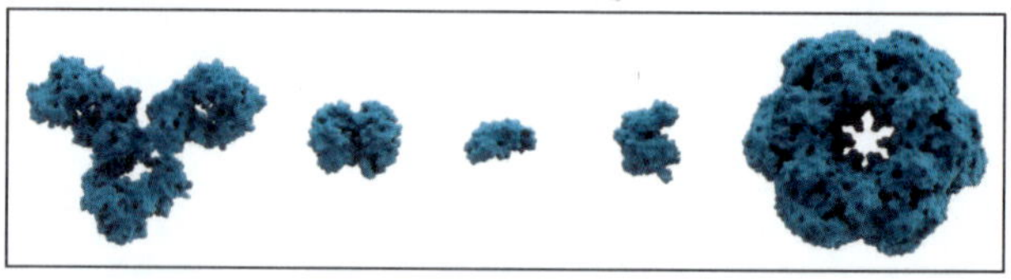

Molecular surface of several proteins showing their comparative sizes. From left to right are: immunoglobulin G (IgG, an antibody), hemoglobin, insulin (a hormone), adenylate kinase (an enzyme), and glutamine synthetase (an enzyme).

Proteins can be informally divided into three main classes, which correlate with typical tertiary structures: globular proteins, fibrous proteins, and membrane proteins. Almost all globular proteins are soluble and many are enzymes. Fibrous proteins are often structural, such as collagen, the major component of connective tissue, or keratin, the protein component of hair and nails. Membrane proteins often serve as receptors or provide channels for polar or charged molecules to pass through the cell membrane.

A special case of intramolecular hydrogen bonds within proteins, poorly shielded from water attack and hence promoting their own dehydration, are called dehydrons.

Protein Domains

Many proteins are composed of several protein domains, i.e. segments of a protein that fold into distinct structural units. Domains usually also have specific functions, such as enzymatic activities (e.g. kinase) or they serve as binding modules (e.g. the SH3 domain binds to proline-rich sequences in other proteins).

Sequence Motif

Short amino acid sequences within proteins often act as recognition sites for other proteins. For instance, SH3 domains typically bind to short PxxP motifs (i.e. 2 prolines [P], separated by 2 unspecified amino acids [x], although the surrounding amino acids may determine the exact binding specificity). A large number of such motifs has been collected in the Eukaryotic Linear Motif (ELM) database.

Cellular Functions

Proteins are the chief actors within the cell, said to be carrying out the duties specified by the information encoded in genes. With the exception of certain types of RNA, most other biological molecules are relatively inert elements upon which proteins act. Proteins make up half the dry weight of an *Escherichia coli* cell, whereas other macromolecules such as DNA and RNA make up only 3% and 20%, respectively. The set of proteins expressed in a particular cell or cell type is known as its proteome.

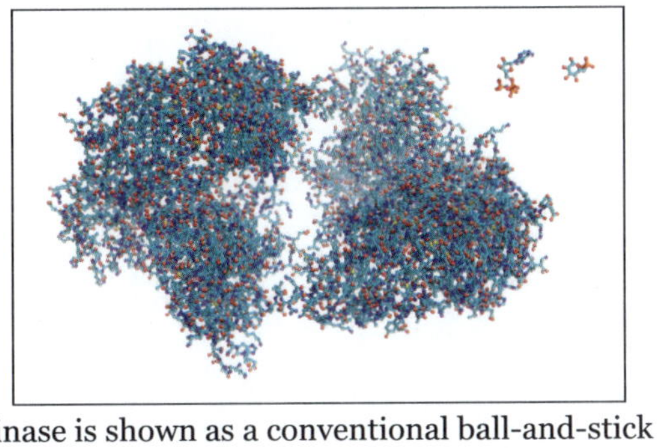

The enzyme hexokinase is shown as a conventional ball-and-stick molecular model. To scale in the top right-hand corner are two of its substrates, ATP and glucose.

The chief characteristic of proteins that also allows their diverse set of functions is their ability to bind other molecules specifically and tightly. The region of the protein responsible for binding another molecule is known as the binding site and is often a depression or "pocket" on the molecular surface. This binding ability is mediated by the tertiary structure of the protein, which defines the binding site pocket, and by the chemical properties of the surrounding amino acids' side chains. Protein binding can be extraordinarily tight and specific; for example, the ribonuclease inhibitor protein binds to human angiogenin with a sub-femtomolar dissociation constant ($<10^{-15}$ M) but does not bind at all to its amphibian homolog onconase (>1 M). Extremely minor chemical changes such as the addition of a single methyl group to a binding partner can sometimes suffice to nearly eliminate binding; for example, the aminoacyl tRNA synthetase specific to the amino acid valine discriminates against the very similar side chain of the amino acid isoleucine.

Proteins can bind to other proteins as well as to small-molecule substrates. When proteins bind specifically to other copies of the same molecule, they can oligomerize to form fibrils; this process occurs often in structural proteins that consist of globular monomers that self-associate to form rigid fibers. Protein–protein interactions also regulate enzymatic activity, control progression through the cell cycle, and allow the assembly of large protein complexes that carry out many closely related reactions with a common biological function. Proteins can also bind to, or even be integrated into, cell membranes. The ability of binding partners to induce conformational changes in proteins allows the construction of enormously complex signaling networks. As interactions between proteins are reversible, and depend heavily on the availability of different groups of partner proteins to form aggregates that are capable to carry out discrete sets of function, study of the interactions between specific proteins is a key to understand important aspects of cellular function, and ultimately the properties that distinguish particular cell types.

Enzymes

The best-known role of proteins in the cell is as enzymes, which catalyse chemical reactions. Enzymes are usually highly specific and accelerate only one or a few chemical reactions. Enzymes carry out most of the reactions involved in metabolism, as well as manipulating DNA in processes such as DNA replication, DNA repair, and transcription. Some enzymes act on other proteins to add or remove chemical groups in a process known as posttranslational modification. About 4,000 reactions are known to be catalysed by enzymes. The rate acceleration conferred by enzymatic catalysis is often enormous—as much as 10^{17}-fold increase in rate over the uncatalysed reaction in the case of orotate decarboxylase (78 million years without the enzyme, 18 milliseconds with the enzyme).

The molecules bound and acted upon by enzymes are called substrates. Although enzymes can consist of hundreds of amino acids, it is usually only a small fraction of the residues that come in contact with the substrate, and an even smaller fraction—three to four residues on average—that are directly involved in catalysis. The region of the enzyme that binds the substrate and contains the catalytic residues is known as the active site.

Dirigent proteins are members of a class of proteins that dictate the stereochemistry of a compound synthesized by other enzymes.

Cell Signaling and Ligand Binding

Many proteins are involved in the process of cell signaling and signal transduction. Some proteins, such as insulin, are extracellular proteins that transmit a signal from the cell in which they were synthesized to other cells in distant tissues. Others are membrane proteins that act as receptors whose main function is to bind a signaling molecule and induce a biochemical response in the cell. Many receptors have a binding site exposed on the cell surface and an effector domain within the cell, which may have enzymatic activity or may undergo a conformational change detected by other proteins within the cell.

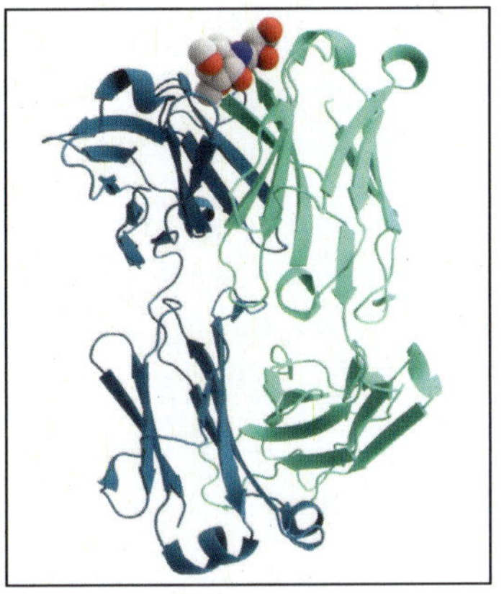

Ribbon diagram of a mouse antibody against cholera that binds a carbohydrate antigen.

Antibodies are protein components of an adaptive immune system whose main function is to bind antigens, or foreign substances in the body, and target them for destruction. Antibodies can be secreted into the extracellular environment or anchored in the membranes of specialized B cells known as plasma cells. Whereas enzymes are limited in their binding affinity for their substrates by the necessity of conducting their reaction, antibodies have no such constraints. An antibody's binding affinity to its target is extraordinarily high.

Many ligand transport proteins bind particular small biomolecules and transport them to other locations in the body of a multicellular organism. These proteins must have a high binding affinity when their ligand is present in high concentrations, but must also release the ligand when it is present at low concentrations in the target tissues. The ca-nonical example of a ligand-binding protein is haemoglobin, which transports oxygen from the lungs to other organs and tissues in all vertebrates and has close homologs in every biological kingdom. Lectins are sugar-binding proteins which are highly specific for their sugar moieties. Lectins typically play a role in biological recognition phenom-ena involving cells and proteins. Receptors and hormones are highly specific binding proteins.

Transmembrane proteins can also serve as ligand transport proteins that alter the permeability of the cell membrane to small molecules and ions. The membrane alone has a hydrophobic core through which polar or charged molecules cannot diffuse. Membrane proteins contain internal channels that allow such molecules to enter and exit the cell. Many ion channel proteins are specialized to select for only a particular ion; for example, potassium and sodium channels often discriminate for only one of the two ions.

Structural Proteins

Structural proteins confer stiffness and rigidity to otherwise-fluid biological components. Most structural proteins are fibrous proteins; for example, collagen and elastin are critical components of connective tissue such as cartilage, and keratin is found in hard or filamentous structures such as hair, nails, feathers, hooves, and some animal shells. Some globular proteins can also play structural functions, for example, actin and tubulin are globular and soluble as monomers, but polymerize to form long, stiff fibers that make up the cytoskeleton, which allows the cell to maintain its shape and size.

Other proteins that serve structural functions are motor proteins such as myosin, kinesin, and dynein, which are capable of generating mechanical forces. These proteins are crucial for cellular motility of single celled organisms and the sperm of many multicellular organisms which reproduce sexually. They also generate the forces exerted by contracting muscles and play essential roles in intracellular transport.

Methods of Study

The activities and structures of proteins may be examined in vitro, in vivo, and in silico. In vitro studies of purified proteins in controlled environments are useful for learning how a protein carries out its function: for example, enzyme kinetics studies explore the chemical mechanism of an enzyme's catalytic activity and its relative affinity for various possible substrate molecules. By contrast, in vivo experiments can provide information about the physiological role of a protein in the context of a cell or even a whole organism. In silico studies use computational methods to study proteins.

Protein Purification

To perform *in vitro* analysis, a protein must be purified away from other cellular components. This process usually begins with cell lysis, in which a cell's membrane is disrupted and its internal contents released into a solution known as a crude lysate. The resulting mixture can be purified using ultracentrifugation, which fractionates the various cellular components into fractions containing soluble proteins; membrane lipids and proteins; cellular organelles, and nucleic acids. Precipitation by a method known as salting out can concentrate the proteins from this lysate. Various types of chromatography are then used to isolate the protein or proteins of interest based on properties such as molecular weight, net charge and binding affinity. The level of purification can be monitored using various types of gel electrophoresis if the desired protein's molecular weight and isoelectric point are known, by spectroscopy if the protein has distinguishable spectroscopic features, or by enzyme assays if the protein has enzymatic activity. Additionally, proteins can be isolated according to their charge using electrofocusing.

For natural proteins, a series of purification steps may be necessary to obtain protein sufficiently pure for laboratory applications. To simplify this process, genetic engineering is often used to add chemical features to proteins that make them easier to purify without affecting their structure or activity. Here, a "tag" consisting of a specific amino acid sequence, often a series of histidine residues (a "His-tag"), is attached to one terminus of the protein. As a result, when the lysate is passed over a chromatography column containing nickel, the histidine residues ligate the nickel and attach to the column while the untagged components of the lysate pass unimpeded. A number of different tags have been developed to help researchers purify specific proteins from complex mixtures.

Cellular Localization

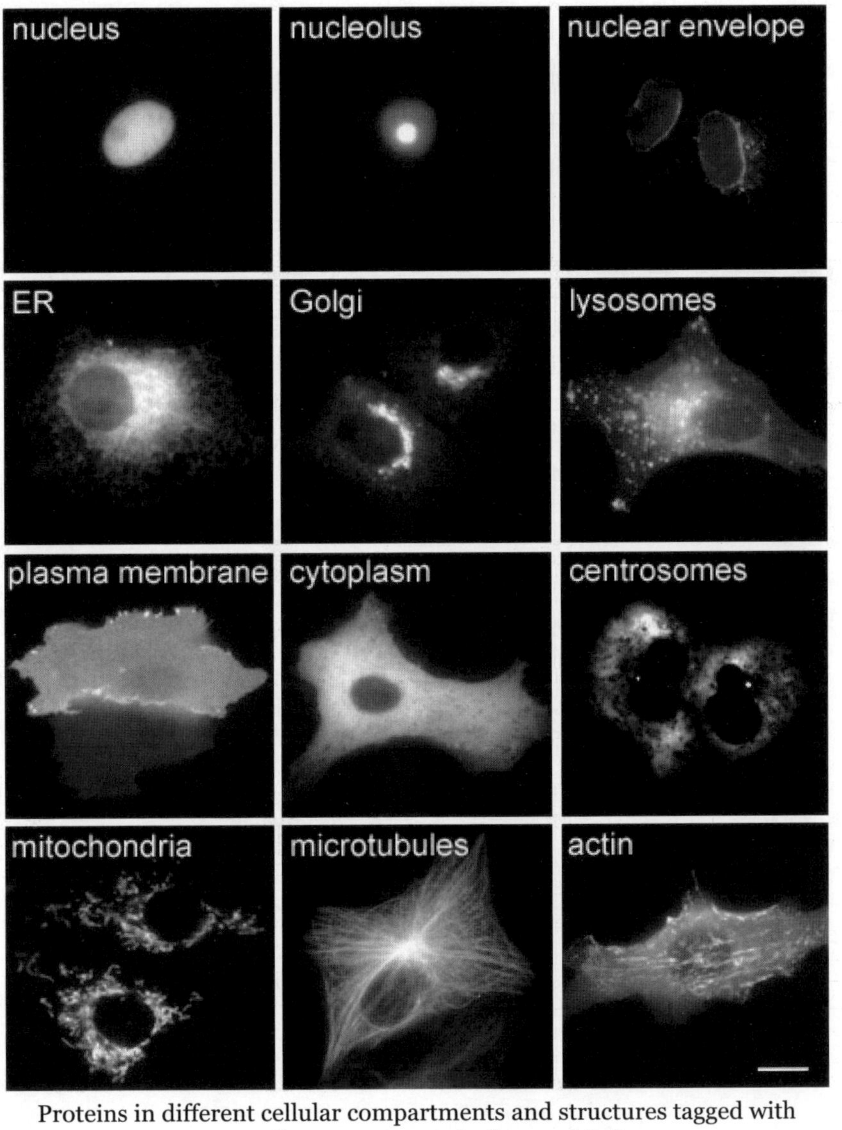

Proteins in different cellular compartments and structures tagged with green fluorescent protein (here, white).

The study of proteins *in vivo* is often concerned with the synthesis and localization of the protein within the cell. Although many intracellular proteins are synthesized in the cytoplasm and membrane-bound or secreted proteins in the endoplasmic reticulum, the specifics of how proteins are targeted to specific organelles or cellular structures is often unclear. A useful technique for assessing cellular localization uses genetic engineering to express in a cell a fusion protein or chimera consisting of the natural protein of interest linked to a "reporter" such as green fluorescent protein (GFP). The fused protein's position within the cell can be cleanly and efficiently visualized using microscopy.

Other methods for elucidating the cellular location of proteins requires the use of known compartmental markers for regions such as the ER, the Golgi, lysosomes or vacuoles, mitochondria, chloroplasts, plasma membrane, etc. With the use of fluorescently tagged versions of these markers or of antibodies to known markers, it becomes much simpler to identify the localization of a protein of interest. For example, indirect immunofluorescence will allow for fluorescence colocalization and demonstration of location. Fluorescent dyes are used to label cellular compartments for a similar purpose.

Other possibilities exist, as well. For example, immunohistochemistry usually utilizes an antibody to one or more proteins of interest that are conjugated to enzymes yielding either luminescent or chromogenic signals that can be compared between samples, allowing for localization information. Another applicable technique is cofractionation in sucrose (or other material) gradients using isopycnic centrifugation. While this technique does not prove colocalization of a compartment of known density and the protein of interest, it does increase the likelihood, and is more amenable to large-scale studies.

Finally, the gold-standard method of cellular localization is immunoelectron microscopy. This technique also uses an antibody to the protein of interest, along with classical electron microscopy techniques. The sample is prepared for normal electron microscopic examination, and then treated with an antibody to the protein of interest that is conjugated to an extremely electro-dense material, usually gold. This allows for the localization of both ultrastructural details as well as the protein of interest.

Through another genetic engineering application known as site-directed mutagenesis, researchers can alter the protein sequence and hence its structure, cellular localization, and susceptibility to regulation. This technique even allows the incorporation of unnatural amino acids into proteins, using modified tRNAs, and may allow the rational design of new proteins with novel properties.

Proteomics

The total complement of proteins present at a time in a cell or cell type is known as its proteome, and the study of such large-scale data sets defines the field of proteomics, named by analogy to the related field of genomics. Key experimental techniques in proteomics include 2D electrophoresis, which allows the separation of a large number of proteins, mass spectrometry, which allows rapid high-throughput identification of proteins and sequencing of peptides (most often after in-gel digestion), protein microarrays, which allow the detection of the relative levels of a large number of proteins present in a cell, and two-hybrid screening, which allows the systematic exploration of protein–protein interactions. The total complement of biologically possible such interactions is known as the interactome. A systematic attempt to determine the structures of proteins representing every possible fold is known as structural genomics.

Bioinformatics

A vast array of computational methods have been developed to analyze the structure, function, and evolution of proteins.

The development of such tools has been driven by the large amount of genomic and proteomic data available for a variety of organisms, including the human genome. It is simply impossible to study all proteins experimentally, hence only a few are subjected to laboratory experiments while computational tools are used to extrapolate to similar proteins. Such homologous proteins can be efficiently identified in distantly related organisms by sequence alignment. Genome and gene sequences can be searched by a variety of tools for certain properties. Sequence profiling tools can find restriction enzyme sites, open reading frames in nucleotide sequences, and predict secondary structures. Phylogenetic trees can be constructed and evolutionary hypotheses developed using special software like ClustalW regarding the ancestry of modern organisms and the genes they express. The field of bioinformatics is now indispensable for the analysis of genes and proteins.

Structure Determination

Discovering the tertiary structure of a protein, or the quaternary structure of its complexes, can provide important clues about how the protein performs its function and how it can be affected, i.e. in drug design. As proteins are too small to be seen under a light microscope, other methods have to be employed to determine their structure. Common experimental methods include X-ray crystallography and NMR spectroscopy, both of which can produce structural information at atomic resolution. However, NMR experiments are able to provide information from which a subset of distances between pairs of atoms can be estimated, and the final possible conformations for a protein are determined by solving a distance geometry problem. Dual polarisation interferometry is a quantitative analytical method for measuring the overall protein conformation and conformational changes due to interactions or other stimulus. Circular dichroism is another laboratory technique for determining internal β-sheet / α-helical composition of proteins. Cryoelectron microscopy is used to produce lower-resolution structural information about very large protein complexes, including assembled viruses; a variant known as electron crystallography can also produce high-resolution information in some cases, especially for two-dimensional crystals of membrane proteins. Solved structures are usually deposited in the Protein Data Bank (PDB), a freely available resource from which structural data about thousands of proteins can be obtained in the form of Cartesian coordinates for each atom in the protein.

Many more gene sequences are known than protein structures. Further, the set of solved structures is biased toward proteins that can be easily subjected to the conditions required in X-ray crystallography, one of the major structure determination methods. In particular, globular proteins are comparatively easy to crystallize in preparation for X-ray crystallography. Membrane proteins and large protein complexes, by contrast, are difficult to crystallize and are underrepresented in the PDB. Structural genomics initiatives have attempted to remedy these deficiencies by systematically solving representative structures of major fold classes. Protein structure prediction methods attempt to provide a means of generating a plausible structure for proteins whose structures have not been experimentally determined.

Structure Prediction and Simulation

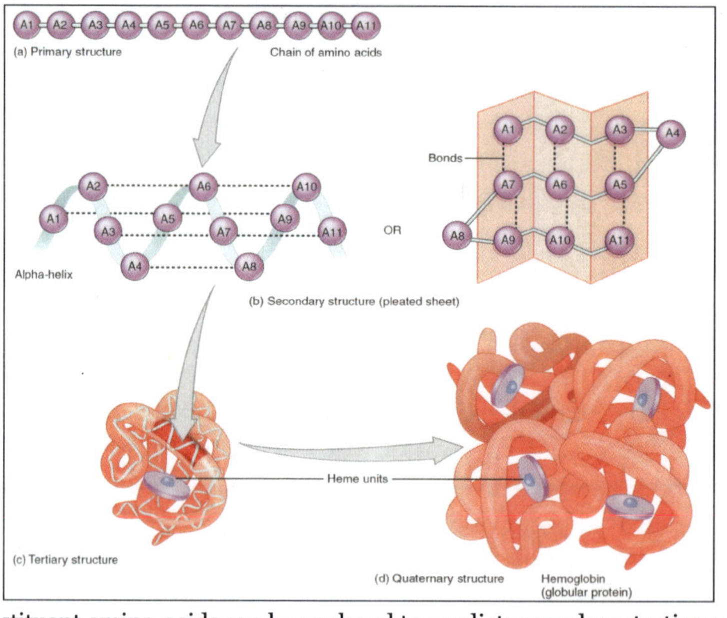

Constituent amino-acids can be analyzed to predict secondary, tertiary and quaternary protein structure, in this case hemoglobin containing heme units.

Complementary to the field of structural genomics, *protein structure prediction* develops efficient mathematical models of proteins to computationally predict the molecular formations in theory, instead of detecting structures with laboratory observation. The most successful type of structure prediction, known as homology modeling, relies on the existence of a "template" structure with sequence similarity to the protein being modeled; structural genomics' goal is to provide sufficient representation in solved structures to model most of those that remain. Although producing accurate models remains a challenge when only distantly related template structures are available, it has been suggested that sequence alignment is the bottleneck in this process, as quite accurate models can be produced if a "perfect" sequence alignment is known. Many structure prediction methods have served to inform the emerging field of protein engineering, in which novel protein folds have already been designed. A more complex computational problem is the prediction of intermolecular interactions, such as in molecular docking and protein–protein interaction prediction.

Mathematical models to simulate dynamic processes of protein folding and binding involve molecular mechanics, in particular, molecular dynamics. Monte Carlo techniques facilitate the computations, which exploit advances in parallel and distributed computing (for example, the Folding@home project which performs molecular modeling on GPUs). *In silico* simulations discovered the folding of small α-helical protein domains such as the villin headpiece and the HIV accessory protein. Hybrid methods combining standard molecular dynamics with quantum mechanical mathematics explored the electronic states of rhodopsins.

Protein Disorder and Unstructure Prediction

Many proteins (in Eucaryota ~33%) contain large unstructured but biologically functional segments and can be classified as intrinsically disordered proteins. Predicting and analysing protein disorder is, therefore, an important part of protein structure characterisation.

Nutrition

Most microorganisms and plants can biosynthesize all 20 standard amino acids, while animals (including humans) must obtain some of the amino acids from the diet. The amino acids that an organism cannot synthesize on its own are referred to as essential amino acids. Key enzymes that synthesize certain amino acids are not present in animals—such as aspartokinase, which catalyses the first step in the synthesis of lysine, methionine, and threonine from aspartate. If amino acids are present in the environment, microorganisms can conserve energy by taking up the amino acids from their surroundings and downregulating their biosynthetic pathways.

In animals, amino acids are obtained through the consumption of foods containing protein. Ingested proteins are then broken down into amino acids through digestion, which typically involves denaturation of the protein through exposure to acid and hydrolysis by enzymes called proteases. Some ingested amino acids are used for protein biosynthesis, while others are converted to glucose through gluconeogenesis, or fed into the citric acid cycle. This use of protein as a fuel is particularly important under starvation conditions as it allows the body's own proteins to be used to support life, particularly those found in muscle.

In animals such as dogs and cats, protein maintains the health and quality of the skin by promoting hair follicle growth and keratinization, and thus reducing the likelihood of skin problems producing malodours. Poor-quality proteins also have a role regarding gastrointestinal health, increasing the potential for flatulence and odorous compounds in dogs because when proteins reach the colon in an undigested state, they are fermented producing hydrogen sulfide gas, indole, and skatole. Dogs and cats digest animal proteins better than those from plants but products of low-quality animal origin are poorly digested, including skin, feathers, and connective tissue.

Protein Metabolism

Protein metabolism denotes the various biochemical processes responsible for the synthesis of proteins and amino acids (anabolism), and the breakdown of proteins by catabolism.

The steps of protein synthesis include transcription, translation, and post translational modifications. During transcription, RNA polymerase transcribes a coding region of the DNA in a cell producing a sequence of RNA, specifically messenger RNA (mRNA). This mRNA sequence contains codons: 3 nucleotide long segments that code for a specific amino acid. Ribosomes translate the codons to their respective amino acids. In humans, non-essential amino acids are synthesized from intermediates in major metabolic pathways such as the Citric Acid Cycle. Essential amino acids must be consumed and are made in other organisms. The amino acids are joined by peptide bonds making a polypeptide chain. This polypeptide chain then goes through post translational modifications and is sometimes joined with other polypeptide chains to form a fully functional protein.

Dietary proteins are first broken down to individual amino acids by various enzymes and hydrochloric acid present in the gastrointestinal tract. These amino acids are further broken down to α-keto acids which can be recycled in the body for generation of energy, and production of glucose or fat or other amino acids. Proteins can be broken down by enzymes known as peptidases or can break down as a result of denaturation. Proteins can denature in environmental conditions the protein is not made for.

Protein Synthesis

Protein anabolism is the process by which protein are formed from amino acids. It relies on five processes: amino acid synthesis, transcription, translation, post translational modifications, and protein folding. Proteins are made from amino acids. In humans, some amino acids can be synthesized using already existing intermediates. These amino acids are known as non-essential amino acids. Essential amino acids require intermediates not present in the human body. These intermediates must be ingested, mostly from eating other organisms.

Amino Acid Synthesis

Pathways that form each amino acid		
Amino Acid	R-group	Pathway
Glycine	H-	Serine + THF → Glycine (hydroxymethyltransferase)
Alanine	CH_3-	Pyruvate → Alanine (aminotransferase)

Valine	$(CH_3)_2$-CH-	Hydroxyethyl-TPP + Pyruvate → α-acetolactate → Valine
Leucine	$(CH_3)_2$-CH-CH_2-	Hydroxyethyl-TPP + Pyruvate → α-ketobutyrate → Leucine
Isoleucine	CH_3-CH_2-CH(CH_3)-	Hydroxyethyl-TPP + Pyruvate → α-acetolactate → Isoleucine
Methionine	CH_3-S-$(CH_2)_2$-	Homocysteine → Methionine (methionine synthase)
Proline	-$(CH_2)_3$-	Glutamic Acid → Glutamate-5-semialdehyde → Proline (γ-glutamyl kinase)
Phenylalanine	Ph-CH_2-	Phosphoenolpyruvate → 2-keto-3-deoxy arabino heptu-losonate-7-phosphate → Chorismate → Phenylalanine
Tryptophan	Ph-NH-CH=C-CH_2-	Phosphoenolpyruvate → 2-keto-3-deoxy arabino heptu-losonate-7-phosphate → Chorismate → Tryptophan
Tyrosine	HO-Ph-CH_2-	Phenylalanine → Tyrosine (phenylalanine hydroxylase)
Serine	HO-CH_2-	3-phosphoglycerate → 3-phosphohydroxypyruvate (3-phosphoglycerate dehydrogenase) → 3-phosphoser-ine (aminotransferase) → Serine (phosphoserine phosphatase)
Threonine	CH_3-CH(OH)-	Aspartate → β-aspartate-semialdehyde → Homoserine → Threonine
Cysteine	HS-CH_2-	Serine → Cystathionine → α-ketobutyrate → Cysteine
Asparagine	H_2N-CO-CH_2-	Aspartic Acid → Asparagine (asparagine synthetase)
Glutamine	H_2N-CO-$(CH_2)_2$-	Glutamic Acid → Glutamine (glutamine synthetase)
Arginine	^+H_2N=C(NH_2)-NH-$(CH_2)_3$-	Glutamate → Glutamate-5-semialdehyde (γ-glutamyl ki-nase) → Arginine
Histidine	NH-CH=N-CH=C-CH_2-	Glucose → Glucose-6-phosphate → Ribose-5-phosphate → Histidine
Lysine	^+H_3N-$(CH_2)_4$-	Aspartate → β-aspartate-semialdehyde → Homoserine + lysine
Aspartic Acid	$^-$OOC-CH_2-	Oxaloacetate → Aspartic Acid (aminotransferase)
Glutamic Acid	$^-$OOC-$(CH_2)_2$-	α-ketoglutarate → Glutamic Acid (aminotransferase)

Polypeptide Synthesis

Transcription

In transcription, RNA polymerase reads a DNA strand and produces an mRNA strand that can be further translated. In order to initiate transcription, the DNA segment that is to be transcribed must be accessible (i.e. it cannot be tightly packed). Once the DNA segment is accessible, the RNA polymerase can begin to transcribe the coding DNA strand by pairing RNA nucleotides to the template DNA strand. During the initial transcription phase, the RNA polymerase searches for a promoter region on the DNA template strand. Once the RNA polymerase binds to this region, it begins to "read" the template DNA strand in the 3' to 5' direction. RNA polymerase attaches RNA bases complementary to the template DNA strand (Uracil will be used instead of Thymine). The new nucleotide bases are bonded to each other covalently. The new bases eventually dissociate from the DNA bases but stay linked to each other, forming a new mRNA strand. This mRNA strand is synthesized in the 5' to 3' direction. Once the RNA reaches a terminator sequence, it dissociates from the DNA template strand and terminates the mRNA sequence as well.

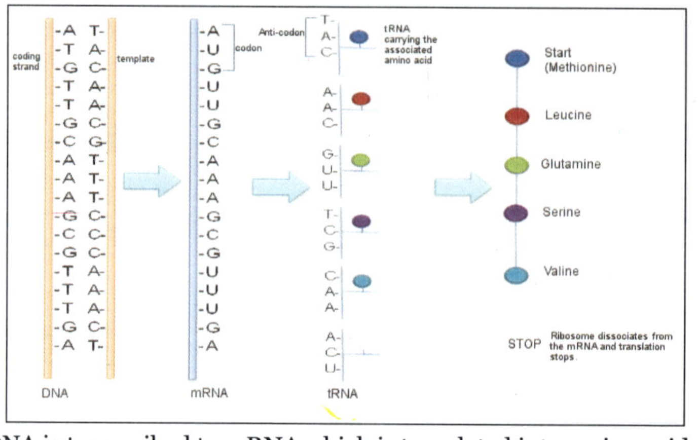

DNA is transcribed to mRNA which is translated into amino acids.

Transcription is regulated in the cell via transcription factors. Transcription factors are proteins that bind to regulatory sequences in the DNA strand such as promoter regions or operator regions. Proteins bound to these regions can either directly halt or allow RNA polymerase to read the DNA strand or can signal other proteins to halt or allow RNA polymerase reading.

Translation

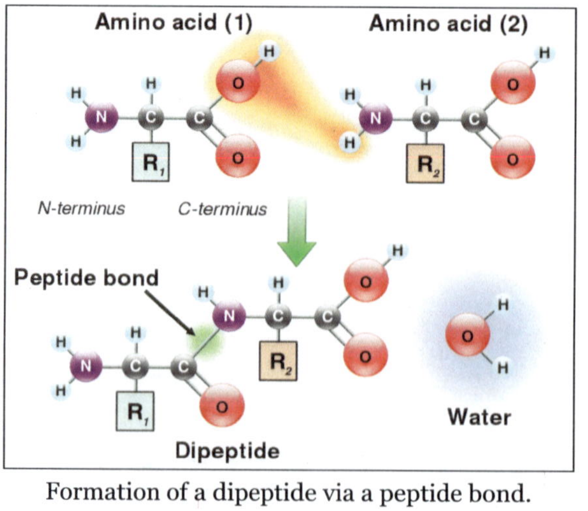

Formation of a dipeptide via a peptide bond.

During translation, ribosomes convert a sequence of mRNA (messenger RNA) to an amino acid sequence. Each 3-base-pair-long segment of mRNA is a codon which corresponds to one amino acid or stop signal. Amino acids can have multiple codons that correspond to them. Ribosomes do not directly attach amino acids to mRNA codons. They must utilize tRNAs (transfer RNAs) as well. Transfer RNAs can bind to amino acids and contain an anticodon which can hydrogen bind to an mRNA codon. The process of bind an amino acid to a tRNA is known as tRNA charging. Here, the enzyme aminoacyl-tRNA-synthetase catalyzes two reactions. In the first one, it attaches an AMP molecule (cleaved from ATP) to the amino acid. The second reaction cleaves the aminoacyl-AMP producing the energy to join the amino acid to the tRNA molecule.

Ribosomes have two subunits, one large and one small. These subunits surround the mRNA strand. The larger subunit contains three binding sites: A (aminoacyl), P (peptidyl), and E (exit). After translational initiation (which is different in prokaryotes and eukaryotes), the ribosome enters the elongation period which follows a repetitive cycle. First a tRNA with the correct amino acid enters the A site. The ribosome transfers the peptide from the tRNA in the P site to the new amino acid on the tRNA in the A site. The tRNA from the P site will be shifted into the E site where it will be ejected. This continually occurs until the ribosome reaches a stop codon or receives a signal to stop. A peptide bond forms between the amino acid attached to the tRNA in the P site and the amino acid attached to a tRNA in the A site. The formation of a peptide bond requires an input of energy. The two reacting molecules are the alpha amino group of one amino acid and the alpha carboxyl group of the other amino acids. A by-product of this bond formation is the release of water (the amino group donates a proton while the carboxyl group donates a hydroxyl).

Translation can be downregulated by miRNAs (microRNAs). These RNA strands can cleave mRNA strands they are complementary to and will thus stop translation. Translation can also be regulated via helper proteins. For example, a protein called eukaryotic initiation factor-2 (eIF-2) can bind to the smaller subunit of the ribosome, starting translation. When elF-2 is phosphorylated, it cannot bind to the ribosome and translation is halted.

Post-Translational Modifications

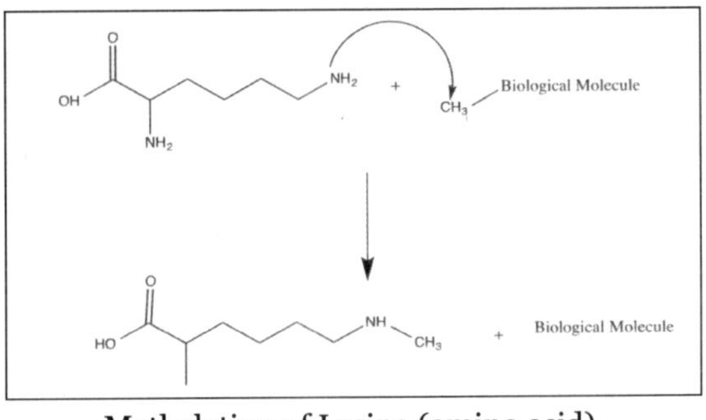

Methylation of Lysine (amino acid).

Once the peptide chain is synthesized, it still must be modified. Post-translational modifications can occur before protein folding or after. Common biological methods of modifying peptide chains after translation include methylation, phosphorylation, and disulfide bond formation. Methylation often occurs to arginine or lysine and involves adding a methyl group to a nitrogen (replacing a hydrogen). The R groups on these amino acids can be methylated multiple times as long as the bonds to nitrogen does not exceed 4. Methylation reduces the ability of these amino acids to form hydrogen bonds so arginine and lysine that are methylated have different properties than their standard counterparts. Phosphorylation often occurs to serine, threonine, and tyrosine and involves replacing a hydrogen on the alcohol group at the terminus of the R group with a phosphate group. This adds a negative charge on the R groups and will thus change how the amino acids behave in comparison to their standard counterparts. Disulfide bond formation is the creation of disulfide bridges (covalent bonds) between two cysteine amino acids in a chain which adds stability to the folded structure.

Protein Folding

A polypeptide chain in the cell does not have to stay linear; it can become branched or fold in on itself. Polypeptide chains fold in a particular manner depending on the solution they are in. The fact that all amino acids contain R groups with different properties is the main reason proteins fold. In a hydrophilic environment such as cytosol, the hydrophobic amino acids will concentrate at the core of the protein, while the hydrophilic amino acids will be on the exterior. This is entropically favorable since water molecules can move much more freely around hydrophilic amino acids than hydrophobic amino acids. In a hydrophobic environment, the hydrophilic amino acids will concentrate at the core of the protein, while the hydrophobic amino acids will be on the exterior. Since the new interactions between the hydrophilic amino acids are stronger than hydrophobic-hydrophilic interactions, this is enthalpically favorable. Once a polypeptide chain is fully folded, it is called a protein. Often many subunits will combine to make a fully functional protein although physiological proteins do exist that contain only one polypeptide chain. Proteins may also incorporate other molecules such as the heme group in hemoglobin, a protein responsible for carrying oxygen in the blood.

Protein Breakdown

Protein catabolism is the process by which proteins are broken down to their amino acids. This is also called proteolysis and can be followed by further amino acid degradation.

Protein Catabolism via Enzymes

Proteases

Originally thought to only disrupt enzymatic reactions, proteases (also known as peptidases) actually help with catabolizing proteins through cleavage and creating new proteins that were not present before. Proteases also help to regulate metabolic pathways. One way they do this is to cleave enzymes in pathways that do not need to be running (i.e. gluconeogenesis when blood glucose concentrations are high). This helps to conserve as much energy as possible and to avoid futile cycles. Futile cycles occur when the catabolic and anabolic pathways are both in effect at the same time and rate for the same reaction. Since the intermediates being created are consumed, the body makes no net gain gains. Energy is lost through futile cycles. Proteases prevent this cycle from occurring by altering the rate of one of the pathways, or by cleaving a key enzyme, they can stop one of the pathways. Proteases are also nonspecific when binding to substrate, allowing for great amounts of diversity inside the cells and other proteins, as they can be cleaved much easier in an energy efficient manner.

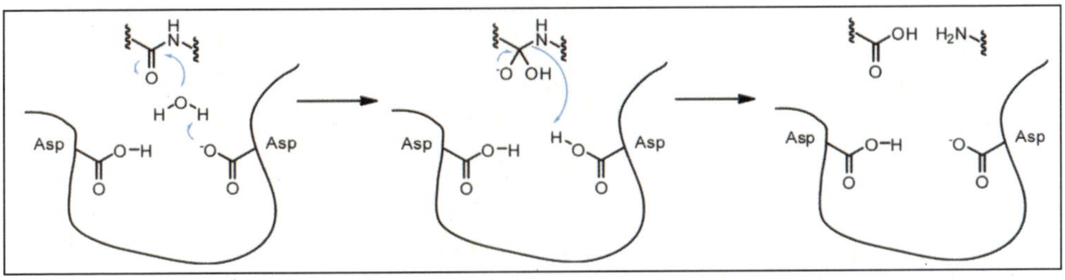

Possible mechanism for Aspartyl Protease cleaving a peptide bond.
Only the peptide bond and active site are shown.

Because many proteases are nonspecific, they are highly regulated in the cell. Without regulation, proteases will destroy many essential proteins for physiological processes. One way the body regulates proteases is through protease inhibitors. Protease inhibitors can be other proteins, small peptides, or molecules. There are two types of protease inhibitors: reversible and irreversible. Reversible protease inhibitors form non-covalent interactions with the protease limiting its functionality. They can be competitive inhibitors, uncompetitive inhibitors, and noncompetitive inhibitors. Competitive inhibitors compete with the peptide to bind to the protease active site. Uncompetitive inhibitors bind to the protease while the peptide is bound but do not let the protease cleave the peptide bond. Noncompetitive inhibitors can do both. Irreversible protease inhibitors covalently modify the active site of the protease so it cannot cleave peptides.

Exopeptidases

Exopeptidases are enzymes that can cleave the end of an amino acid side chain mostly through the addition of water. These enzymes have two classes: aminopeptidases and carboxypeptidases. Aminopeptidases are enzymes that remove amino acids from the amino terminus of protein. They are present in all lifeforms and are crucial for survival since they do many cellular tasks in order to maintain stability. This form of peptidase is a zinc metalloenzyme and it is inhibited by the transition state analog. This analog is similar to the actual transition state, so it can make the enzyme bind to it instead of the actual transition state, thus preventing substrate binding and decreasing reaction rates.

Carboxypeptidases cleave at the carboxyl end of the protein. While they can catabolize proteins, they are more often used in post-transcriptional modifications.

Endopeptidases

Endopeptidases are enzymes that add water to an internal peptide bond in a peptide chain and break that bond. Three common endopeptidases are pepsin, trypsin, and chymotrypsin. Chymotrypsin performs a hydrolysis reaction that cleaves after aromatic residues. The main amino acids involved are serine, histidine, and aspartic acid. They all play a role in cleaving the peptide bond. These three amino acids are known as the catalytic triad which means that these three must all be present in order to properly function. Trypsin cleaves after long positively charged residues and has a negatively charged binding pocket at the active site. Both are produced as zymogens, meaning they are initially found in their inactive state and after cleavage though a hydrolysis reaction, they becomes activated. Non-covalent interactions such as hydrogen bonding between the peptide backbone and the catalytic triad help increase reaction rates, allowing these peptidases to cleave many peptides efficiently.

Protein Catabolism via Environmental Changes

pH

Cellular proteins are held in a relatively constant pH in order to prevent changes in the protonation state of amino acids. If the pH drops, some amino acids in the polypeptide chain can become protonated if the pka of their R groups is higher than the new pH. Protonation can change the charge these R groups have. If the pH raises, some amino acids in the chain can become deprotonated (if the pka of the R group is lower than the new pH). This also changes the R group charge. Since many amino acids interact with other amino acids based on electrostatic attraction, changing the charge can break these interactions. The loss of these interactions alters the proteins structure, but most importantly it alters the proteins function, which can be beneficial or detrimental. A significant change in pH may even disrupt many interactions the amino acids make and denature (unfold) the protein.

Temperature

As the temperature in the environment increases, molecules move faster. Hydrogen bonds and hydrophobic interactions are important stabilizing forces in proteins. If the temperature rises and molecules containing these interactions are moving too fast, the interactions become compromised or even break. At high temperatures, these interactions cannot form, and a functional protein is denatured. However, it relies on two factors; the type of protein used and the amount of heat applied. The amount of heat applied determines whether this change in protein is permanent or if it can be transformed back to its original form.

Fats

Fats are one of the three main macronutrients, along with carbohydrates and proteins. Fat molecules consist of primarily carbon and hydrogen atoms and are therefore hydrophobic and are soluble in organic solvents and insoluble in water. Examples include cholesterol, phospholipids, and triglycerides.

The terms *lipid*, *oil*, and *fat* are often confused. *Lipid* is the general term, though a lipid is not necessarily a triglyceride. *Oil* normally refers to a lipid with short or unsaturated fatty acid chains that is liquid at room temperature, while *fat* (in the strict sense) specifically refers to lipids that are solids at room temperature – however, *fat* (in the broad sense) may be used in food science as a synonym for lipid.

Fat is an important foodstuff for many forms of life, and fats serve both structural and metabolic functions. They are a necessary part of the diet of most heterotrophs (including humans) and are the most energy dense, thus the most efficient form of energy storage.

Some fatty acids that are set free by the digestion of fats are called essential because they cannot be synthesized in the body from simpler constituents. There are two essential fatty acids (EFAs) in human nutrition: alpha-linolenic acid (an omega-3 fatty acid) and linoleic acid (an omega-6 fatty acid). Other lipids needed by the body can be synthesized from these and other fats. Fats and other lipids are broken down in the body by enzymes called lipases produced in the pancreas.

Fats and oils are categorized according to the number and bonding of the carbon atoms in the aliphatic chain. Fats that are saturated fats have no double bonds between the carbons in the chain. Unsaturated fats have one or more double bonded carbons in the chain. The nomenclature is based on the non-acid (non-carbonyl) end of the chain. This end is called the omega end or the n-end. Thus alpha-linolenic acid is called an omega-3 fatty acid because the 3rd carbon from that end is the first double bonded carbon in the chain counting from that end. Some oils and fats have multiple double bonds and are therefore called polyunsaturated fats. Unsaturated fats can be further divided into cis fats, which are the most common in nature, and trans fats, which are rare in nature. Unsaturated fats can be altered by reaction with hydrogen effected by a catalyst. This action, called hydrogenation, tends to break all the double bonds and makes a fully saturated fat. To make vegetable shortening, then, liquid *cis*-unsaturated fats such as vegetable oils are hydrogenated to produce saturated fats, which have more desirable physical properties e.g., they melt at a desirable temperature (30–40 °C), and store well, whereas polyunsaturated oils go rancid when they react with oxygen in the air. However, trans fats are generated during hydrogenation as contaminants created by an unwanted side reaction on the catalyst during partial hydrogenation.

Saturated fats can stack themselves in a closely packed arrangement, so they can solidify easily and are typically solid at room temperature. For example, animal fats tallow and lard are high in saturated fatty acid content and are solids. Olive and linseed oils on the other hand are unsaturated and liquid. Fats serve both as energy sources for the body, and as stores for energy in excess of what the body needs immediately. Each gram of fat when burned or metabolized releases about 9 food calories (37 kJ = 8.8 kcal). Fats are broken down in the healthy body to release their constituents, glycerol and fatty acids. Glycerol itself can be converted to glucose by the liver and so become a source of energy.

Chemical Structure

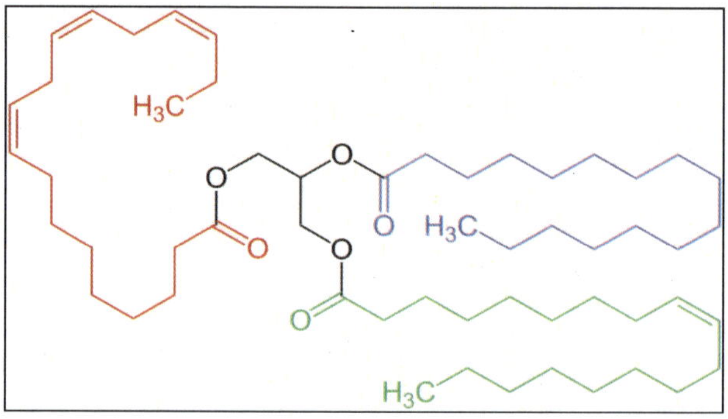

Example of a natural triglyceride with three different fatty acids. One fatty acid is saturated (blue highlighted), another contains one double bond within the carbon chain (green highlighted). The third fatty acid (a polyunsaturated fatty acid, highlighted in red) contains three double bonds within the carbon chain. All carbon-carbon double bonds shown are *cis* isomers.

There are many different kinds of fats, but each is a variation on the same chemical structure. All fats are derivatives of fatty acids and glycerol. Most fats are glycerides, particularly triglycerides (triesters of glycerol). One chain of fatty acid is bonded to each of the three -OH groups of the glycerol by the reaction of the carboxyl end of the fatty acid (-COOH) with the alcohol; I.e. three chains per molecule. Water is eliminated and the carbons are linked by an -O- bond through dehydration synthesis. This process is called esterification and fats are therefore esters. As a simple visual illustration, if the kinks and angles of these chains were straightened out, the molecule would have the shape of a capital letter E. The fatty acids would each be a horizontal line; the glycerol "backbone" would be the vertical line that joins the horizontal lines. Fats therefore have "ester" bonds.

The properties of any specific fat molecule depend on the particular fatty acids that constitute it. Fatty acids form a family of compounds that are composed of increasing numbers of carbon atoms linked into a zig-zag chain (hydrogen atoms to the side). The more carbon atoms there are in any fatty acid, the longer its chain will be. Long chains are more susceptible to intermolecular forces of attraction (in this case, van der Waals forces), and so the longer ones melt at a higher temperature (melting point).

Examples of Fatty Acids.		
Trans Unsaturated (Example Shown: Elaidic acid)	Cis Unsaturated (Example shown: Oleic acid)	Saturated (Example shown: Stearic acid)
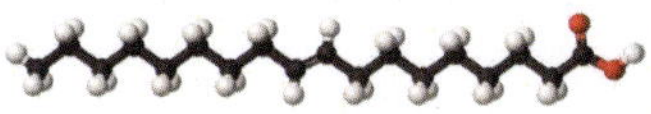	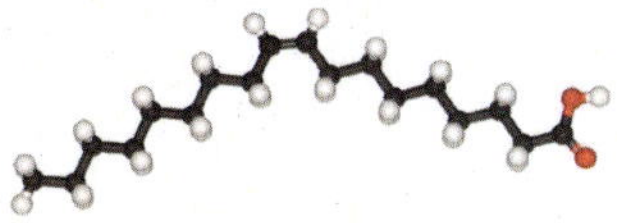	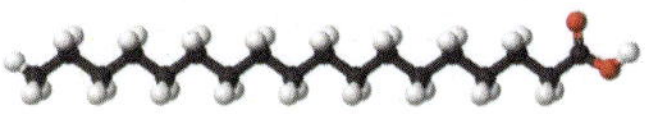
Elaidic acid is the principal trans unsaturated fatty acid often found in partially hydrogenated vegetable oils.	Oleic acid is a cis unsaturated fatty acid making up 55–80% of olive oil.	Stearic acid is a saturated fatty acid found in animal fats and is the intended product in full hydrogenation. Stearic acid is neither cis nor trans because it has no carbon-carbon double bonds.

Fatty acid chains may also differ by length, often categorized as short to very long.

- Short-chain fatty acids (SCFA) are fatty acids with aliphatic tails of fewer than six carbons (i.e. butyric acid).
- Medium-chain fatty acids (MCFA) are fatty acids with aliphatic tails of 6–12 carbons, which can form medium-chain triglycerides.
- Long-chain fatty acids (LCFA) are fatty acids with aliphatic tails of 13 to 21 carbons.
- Very long chain fatty acids (VLCFA) are fatty acids with aliphatic tails of 22 or more carbons.

Any of these aliphatic fatty acid chains may be glycerated and the resultant fats may have tails of different lengths from very short triformin to very long, e.g., cerotic acid, or *hexacosanoic acid*, a 26-carbon long-chain saturated fatty acid. Long chain fats are exemplified by tallow (lard) whose chains are 17 carbons long. Most fats found in food, whether vegetable or animal, are made up of medium to long-chain fatty acids, usually of equal or nearly equal length. Many cell types can use either glucose or fatty acids for this energy. In particular, heart and skeletal muscle prefer fatty acids. Despite long-standing assertions to the contrary, fatty acids can also be used as a source of fuel for brain cells.

Importance for Living Organisms

Fats are also sources of essential fatty acids, an important dietary requirement. They provide energy as noted above. Vitamins A, D, E, and K are fat-soluble, meaning they can only be digested, absorbed, and transported in conjunction with fats. Fats play a vital role in maintaining healthy skin and hair, insulating body organs against shock, maintaining body temperature, and promoting healthy cell function. Fat also serves as a useful buffer against a host of diseases. When a particular substance, whether chemical or biotic, reaches unsafe levels in the bloodstream, the body can effectively dilute—or at least maintain equilibrium of—the offending substances by storing it in new fat tissue. This helps to protect vital organs, until such time as the offending substances can be metabolized or removed from the body by such means as excretion, urination, accidental or intentional bloodletting, sebum excretion, and hair growth.

Adipose Tissue

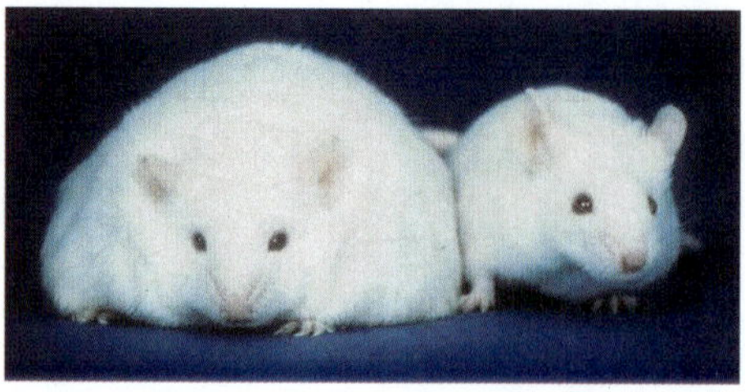

The obese mouse on the left has large stores of adipose tissue. For comparison, a mouse with a normal amount of adipose tissue is shown above.

In animals, adipose tissue, or fatty tissue is the body's means of storing metabolic energy over extended periods of time. Adipocytes (fat cells) store fat derived from the diet and from liver metabolism. Under energy stress these cells may degrade their stored fat to supply fatty acids and also glycerol to the circulation. These metabolic activities are regulated by several hormones (e.g., insulin, glucagon and epinephrine). Adipose tissue also secretes the hormone leptin.

The location of the tissue determines its metabolic profile: visceral fat is located within the abdominal wall (i.e., beneath the wall of abdominal muscle) whereas "subcutaneous fat" is located beneath the skin (and includes fat that is located in the abdominal area beneath the skin but *above* the abdominal muscle wall). Visceral fat was recently discovered to be a significant producer of signaling chemicals (i.e., hormones), among which several are involved in inflammatory tissue responses. One of these is resistin which has been linked to obesity, insulin resistance, and Type 2 diabetes. This latter result is currently controversial, and there have been reputable studies supporting all sides on the issue.

Fatty Acids and Human Health

Dietary consumption of fatty acids has effects on human health. Studies have found that replacing saturated fats with *cis* unsaturated fats in the diet reduces risk of cardiovascular disease. For example, a systematic review of randomized control trials by the Cochrane Library concluded: "Lifestyle advice to all those at risk of cardiovascular disease and to lower risk population groups should continue to include permanent reduction of dietary saturated fat and partial replacement by unsaturated fats."

Numerous studies have also found that consumption of *trans* fats increases risk of cardiovascular disease. The Harvard School of Public Health advises that replacing *trans* fats and saturated fats with *cis* monounsaturated and polyunsaturated fats is beneficial for health. A meta-analyses of randomized controlled trials found that reducing fat and cholesterol intake does not effect cardiovascular disease or all cause mortality.

Fat Metabolism

Fat metabolism refers to the processes involved in the biosynthesis and breakdown of fats. The metabolic break down of dietary fats supports many life-sustaining functions. Metabolized fat is stored as a reserve source of energy for use when needed. Fat provides insulation to keep your body warm; the fat beneath your skin is a source of heat when skin temperature drops. Fat cushions and protects your organs, and, in addition to your liver, fat provides storage for fat-soluble vitamins. The myelin sheath covering in your brain is also made up of 70 percent fat, according to Franklin Institute. Exercise and gender can affect the speed of fat metabolism.

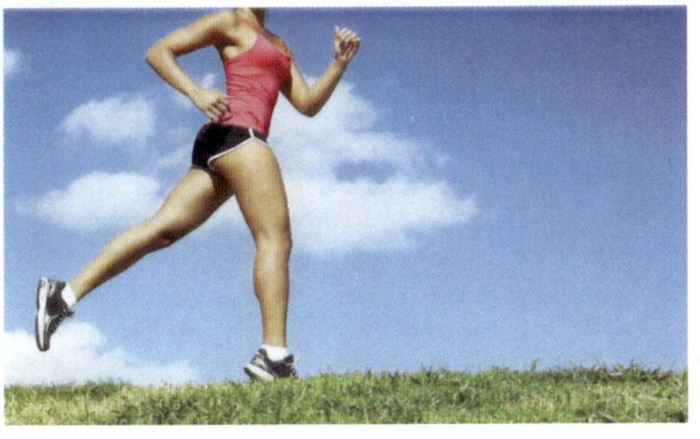

Fat Energy

Fat, or adipose tissue, is your body's largest energy reserve, containing about 100,000 calories. Without additional food, fat can support metabolic functions for 30 to 40 days, according to Dr. Charles E. Ophardt, Professor Emeritus, Elmhurst College. However, water intake must be maintained. Fat molecules, as compared with carbohydrate molecules, contain little water. Based on this fact, Ophardt states, if glycogen, the storage form of carbohydrates, replaced fat stores in a 154-pound male, his body weight would increase by about 110 pounds because of the additional water weight.

The Power Switch

Dietary fat is broken down and stored in your fat cells as triglycerides, which are made up of three fatty acids and glycerol. Several chemicals help move stored fat out of adipose cells and into the blood stream for energy usage. Hormone sensitive lipase, found within the fat cell, and lipoprotein lipase are enzymes that help facilitate the release of fat with the help of the hormone epinephrine. This process is called lipolysis. When stimulated by epinephrine, HSL breaks down stored triglycerides and their components, three free fatty acids and glycerol, and releases them into the blood stream. Exercise enhances the response of HSL to epinephrine and increases fat burning. Obesity decreases HSLs response to epinephrine and slows fat metabolism, according to Len Kravitz, Ph.D., researcher and professor of exercise science at New Mexico University. LPL, found on blood vessel walls, controls how fat is distributed to its storage sites on your body.

References

- Hooper, Lee; Martin, Nicole; Abdelhamid, Asmaa; Davey Smith, George (2015). "Reduction in saturated fat intake for cardiovascular disease". Cochrane Database of Systematic Reviews (6): CD011737. doi:10.1002/14651858.CD011737. PMID 26068959
- Carbohydrates-51976: livescience.com, Retrieved 29 May, 2019
- Koegl M, Uetz P (December 2007). "Improving yeast two-hybrid screening systems". Briefings in Functional Genomics & Proteomics. 6(4): 302–12. doi:10.1093/bfgp/elm035. PMID 18218650
- Voet D, Pratt CW, Voet JG (2013) [2012]. Fundamentals of biochemistry : life at the molecular level (4th ed.). Hoboken, NJ: John Wiley & Sons. pp. 712–765. ISBN 9780470547847. OCLC 782934336
- What-is-fat-metabolism-442981: livestrong.com, Retrieved 19 July, 2019
- López-Otín C, Bond JS (November 2008). "Proteases: multifunctional enzymes in life and disease". The Journal of Biological Chemistry. 283 (45): 30433–7. doi:10.1074/jbc.R800035200. PMC 2576539. PMID 18650443

4
Micronutrients: Vitamins and Minerals

The micronutrients within the body are divided into two broad categories, vitamins and minerals. Some of the different vitamins are vitamin A, B, C, D, E and K. There are a number of minerals which are vital for metabolism such as manganese, calcium and phosphorus. This chapter has been carefully written to provide an easy understanding of these varied micronutrients.

Vitamin

A vitamin is one of a group of organic substances that is present in minute amounts in natural foodstuffs. Vitamins are essential to normal metabolism. If we do not take enough of any kind of vitamin, certain medical conditions can result.

A vitamin is both:

- An organic compound, which means it contains carbon.
- An essential nutrient that body cannot produce enough of and which it needs to get from food.

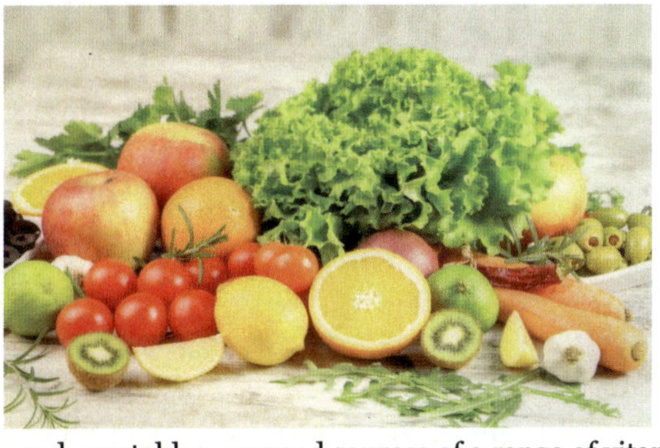

Fruits and vegetables are good sources of a range of vitamins.

Fat-Soluble and Water-soluble Vitamins

Vitamins are either fat-soluble or water-soluble.

Fat-Soluble Vitamins

Fat-soluble vitamins are stored in the fatty tissues of the body and the liver. Vitamins A, D, E, and K are fat-soluble. These are easier to store than water-soluble vitamins, and they can stay in the body as reserves for days, and sometimes months.

Fat-soluble vitamins are absorbed through the intestinal tract with the help of fats, or lipids.

Water-Soluble Vitamins

Water-soluble vitamins do not stay in the body for long. The body cannot store them, and they are soon excreted in urine. Because of this, water-soluble vitamins need to be replaced more often than fat-soluble ones.

Vitamin C and all the B vitamins are water soluble.

Vitamin A

Vitamin A is a group of unsaturated nutritional organic compounds that includes retinol, retinal, retinoic acid, and several provitamin A carotenoids (most notably beta-carotene). Vitamin A has multiple functions: it is important for growth and development, for the maintenance of the immune system and good vision. Vitamin A is needed by the retina of the eye in the form of retinal, which combines with protein opsin to form rhodopsin, the light-absorbing molecule necessary for both low-light (scotopic vision) and color vision. Vitamin A also functions in a very different role as retinoic acid (an irreversibly oxidized form of retinol), which is an important hormone-like growth factor for epithelial and other cells.

In foods of animal origin, the major form of vitamin A is an ester, primarily retinyl palmitate, which is converted to retinol (chemically an alcohol) in the small intestine. The retinol form functions as a storage form of the vitamin, and can be converted to and from its visually active aldehyde form, retinal.

All forms of vitamin A have a beta-ionone ring to which an isoprenoid chain is attached, called a *retinyl group*. Both structural features are essential for vitamin activity. The orange pigment of carrots (beta-carotene) can be represented as two connected retinyl groups, which are used in the body to contribute to vitamin A levels. Alpha-carotene and gamma-carotene also have a single retinyl group, which give them some vitamin activity. None of the other carotenes have vitamin activity. The carotenoid beta-cryptoxanthin possesses an ionone group and has vitamin activity in humans.

Vitamin A can be found in two principal forms in foods:

- Retinol, the form of vitamin A absorbed when eating animal food sources, is a yellow, fat-soluble substance. Since the pure alcohol form is unstable, the vitamin is found in tissues in a form of retinyl ester. It is also commercially produced and administered as esters such as retinyl acetate or palmitate.
- The carotenes alpha-carotene, beta-carotene, gamma-carotene; and the xanthophyll beta-cryptoxanthin (all of which contain beta-ionone rings), but no other carotenoids, function as provitamin A in herbivores and omnivore animals, which possess the enzyme beta-carotene 15,15'-dioxygenase which cleaves beta-carotene in the intestinal mucosa and converts it to retinol.

Deficiency

Vitamin A deficiency is estimated to affect approximately one third of children under the age of five around the world. It is estimated to claim the lives of 670,000 children under five annually. Approximately 250,000–500,000 children in developing countries become blind each year owing to vitamin A deficiency, with the highest prevalence in Southeast Asia and Africa. Vitamin A deficiency is "the leading cause of preventable childhood blindness," according to UNICEF. It also increases the risk of death from common childhood conditions such as diarrhea. UNICEF regards addressing vitamin A deficiency as critical to reducing child mortality, the fourth of the United Nations' Millennium Development Goals.

Vitamin A deficiency can occur as either a primary or a secondary deficiency. A primary vitamin A deficiency occurs among children and adults who do not consume an adequate intake of provitamin A carotenoids from fruits and vegetables or preformed vitamin A from animal and dairy products. Early weaning from breastmilk can also increase the risk of vitamin A deficiency.

Secondary vitamin A deficiency is associated with chronic malabsorption of lipids, impaired bile production and release, and chronic exposure to oxidants, such as cigarette smoke, and chronic alcoholism. Vitamin A is a fat-soluble vitamin and depends on micellar solubilization for dispersion into the small intestine, which results in poor use of vitamin A from low-fat diets. Zinc deficiency can also impair absorption, transport, and metabolism of vitamin A because it is essential for the synthesis of the vitamin A transport proteins and as the cofactor in conversion of retinol to retinal. In malnourished populations, common low intakes of vitamin A and zinc increase the severity of vitamin A deficiency and lead physiological signs and symptoms of deficiency. A study in Burkina Faso showed major reduction of malaria morbidity with combined vitamin A and zinc supplementation in young children.

Due to the unique function of retinal as a visual chromophore, one of the earliest and specific manifestations of vitamin A deficiency is impaired vision, particularly in reduced light – night blindness. Persistent deficiency gives rise to a series of changes, the most devastating of which occur in the eyes. Some other ocular changes are referred to as xerophthalmia. First there is dryness of the conjunctiva (xerosis) as the normal lacrimal and mucus-secreting epithelium is replaced by a keratinized epithelium. This is followed by the build-up of keratin debris in small opaque plaques (Bitot's spots) and, eventually, erosion of the roughened corneal surface with softening and destruction of the cornea (keratomalacia) and leading to total blindness. Other changes include impaired immunity (increased risk of ear infections, urinary tract infections, Meningococcal disease), hyperkeratosis (white lumps at hair follicles), keratosis pilaris and squamous metaplasia of the epithelium lining the upper respiratory passages and urinary bladder to a keratinized epithelium. In relation to dentistry, a deficiency in vitamin A may lead to enamel hypoplasia.

Adequate supply, but not excess vitamin A, is especially important for pregnant and breastfeeding women for normal fetal development and in breastmilk. Deficiencies cannot be compensated by postnatal supplementation. Excess vitamin A, which is most common with high dose vitamin supplements, can cause birth defects and therefore should not exceed recommended daily values.

Vitamin A metabolic inhibition as a result of alcohol consumption during pregnancy is one proposed mechanism for fetal alcohol syndrome and is characterized by teratogenicity resembling maternal vitamin A deficiency or reduced retinoic acid synthesis during embryogenesis.

Vitamin A Supplementation

A review found no evidence that beta-carotene or vitamin A supplements increase longevity in healthy people or in people with various diseases. A review found that vitamin A supplementation of children under five who are at risk of deficiency reduced mortality by up to 24%. However, a Cochrane review concluded there was not evidence to recommend blanket vitamin A supplementation for all infants less than a year of age, as it did not reduce infant mortality or morbidity in low- and middle-income countries. The World Health Organization estimated that vitamin A supplementation averted 1.25 million deaths due to vitamin A deficiency in 40 countries since 1998.

While strategies include intake of vitamin A through a combination of breast feeding and dietary intake, delivery of oral high-dose supplements remain the principal strategy for minimizing deficiency. About 75% of the vitamin A required for supplementation activity by developing countries is supplied by the Micronutrient Initiative with support from the Canadian International Development Agency. Food fortification approaches are feasible, but cannot ensure adequate intake levels. Observational studies of pregnant women in sub-Saharan Africa have shown that low serum vitamin A levels are associated with an increased risk of mother-to-child transmission of HIV. Low blood vitamin A levels have been associated with rapid HIV infection and deaths. Possible mechanisms of HIV transmission found no relationship between blood vitamin A levels in the mother and infant, with conventional intervention established by treatment with anti-HIV drugs.

Side Effects

Since vitamin A is fat-soluble, disposing of any excesses taken in through diet takes much longer than with water-soluble B vitamins and vitamin C. This allows for toxic levels of vitamin A to accumulate. These toxicities only occur with preformed (retinoid) vitamin A (such as from liver). The carotenoid forms (such as beta-carotene as found in carrots), give no such symptoms, but excessive dietary intake of beta-carotene can lead to carotenodermia, a harmless but cosmetically displeasing orange-yellow discoloration of the skin.

In general, acute toxicity occurs at doses of 25,000 IU/kg of body weight, with chronic toxicity occurring at 4,000 IU/kg of body weight daily for 6–15 months. However, liver toxicities can occur at levels as low as 15,000 IU (4500 micrograms) per day to 1.4 million IU per day, with an average daily toxic dose of 120,000 IU, particularly with excessive consumption of alcohol. In people with renal failure, 4000 IU can cause substantial damage. Signs of toxicity may occur with long-term consumption of vitamin A at doses of 25,000–33,000 IU per day.

Excessive vitamin A consumption can lead to nausea, irritability, anorexia (reduced appetite), vomiting, blurry vision, headaches, hair loss, muscle and abdominal pain and weakness, drowsiness, and altered mental status. In chronic cases, hair loss, dry skin, drying of the mucous membranes, fever, insomnia, fatigue, weight loss, bone fractures, anemia, and diarrhea can all be evident on top of the symptoms associated with less serious toxicity. Some of these symptoms are also common to acne treatment with Isotretinoin. Chronically high doses of vitamin A, and also pharmaceutical retinoids such as 13-cis retinoic acid, can produce the syndrome of pseudotumor cerebri. This syndrome includes headache, blurring of vision and confusion, associated with increased intracerebral pressure. Symptoms begin to resolve when intake of the offending substance is stopped.

Chronic intake of 1500 RAE of preformed vitamin A may be associated with osteoporosis and hip fractures because it suppresses bone building while simultaneously stimulating bone breakdown, although other reviews have disputed this effect, indicating further evidence is needed.

A systematic review found that beta-carotene and higher doses of supplemental vitamin A increased mortality in healthy people and people with various diseases. The findings of the review extend evidence that antioxidants may not have long-term benefits.

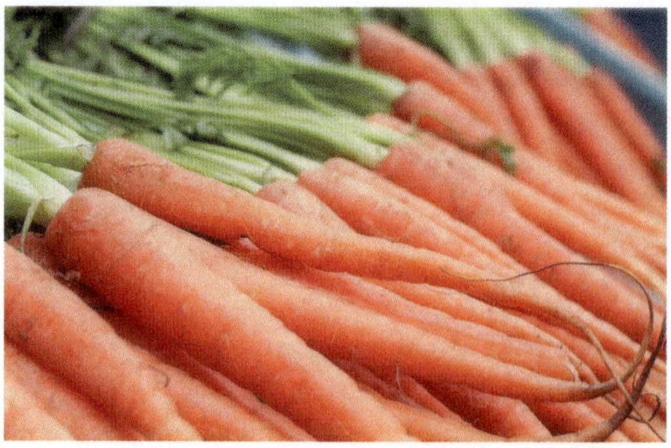

Carrots are a source of beta-carotene.

Vitamin A is found in many foods, including the following list. Bracketed values are retinol activity equivalences (RAEs) and percentage of the adult male RDA, per 100 grams of the foodstuff (average). Conversion of carotene to retinol varies from person to person and bioavailability of carotene in food varies.

Source	Retinol activity equivalences (RAEs) (in µg)	Percentage of the adult male RDA per 100 g of the foodstuff
Cod liver oil	30000	3333%
Liver turkey	8058	895%
Liver beef, pork, fish	6500	722%
Liver chicken	3296	366%
Ghee	3069	344%
Sweet potato	961	107%
Carrot	835	93%
Broccoli leaf	800	89%
Butter	684	76%
Kale	681	76%
Collard greens frozen then boiled	575	64%
Butternut squash	532	67%
Dandelion greens	508	56%
Spinach	469	52%
Pumpkin	426	43%
Collard greens	333	37%
Cheddar cheese	265	29%
Cantaloupe melon	169	19%
Bell pepper/capsicum, red	157	17%
Egg	140	16%
Apricot	96	11%
Papaya	55	6%
Tomatoes	42	5%

Mango	38	4%
Pea	38	4%
Broccoli florets	31	3%
Milk	28	3%
Bell pepper/capsicum, green	18	2%
Spirulina	3	0.3%

Metabolic Functions

Vitamin A plays a role in a variety of functions throughout the body, such as:

- Vision,
- Gene transcription,
- Immune function,
- Embryonic development and reproduction,
- Bone metabolism,
- Haematopoiesis,
- Skin and cellular health,
- Teeth,
- Mucous membrane.

Vision

The role of vitamin A in the visual cycle is specifically related to the retinal form. Within the eye, 11-*cis*-retinal is bound to the protein "opsin" to form rhodopsin in rods and iodopsin (cones) at conserved lysine residues. As light enters the eye, the 11-*cis*-retinal is isomerized to the all-"trans" form. The all-"trans" retinal dissociates from the opsin in a series of steps called photo-bleaching. This isomerization induces a nervous signal along the optic nerve to the visual center of the brain. After separating from opsin, the all-"trans"-retinal is recycled and converted back to the 11-"cis"-retinal form by a series of enzymatic reactions. In addition, some of the all-"trans" retinal may be converted to all-"trans" retinol form and then transported with an interphotoreceptor retinol-binding protein (IRBP) to the pigment epithelial cells. Further esterification into all-"trans" retinyl esters allow for storage of all-trans-retinol within the pigment epithelial cells to be reused when needed. The final stage is conversion of 11-*cis*-retinal will rebind to opsin to reform rhodopsin (visual purple) in the retina. Rhodopsin is needed to see in low light (contrast) as well as for night vision. Kühne showed that rhodopsin in the retina is only regenerated when the retina is attached to retinal pigmented epithelium, which provides retinal. It is for this reason that a deficiency in vitamin A will inhibit the reformation of rhodopsin and lead to one of the first symptoms, night blindness.

Gene Transcription

Vitamin A, in the retinoic acid form, plays an important role in gene transcription. Once retinol has been taken up by a cell, it can be oxidized to retinal (retinaldehyde) by retinol dehydrogenases and then retinaldehyde can be oxidized to retinoic acid by retinaldehyde dehydrogenases. The conversion of retinaldehyde to retinoic acid is an irreversible step, meaning that the production of retinoic acid is tightly regulated, due to its activity as a ligand for nuclear receptors. The physiological form of retinoic acid (all-trans-retinoic acid) regulates gene transcription by binding to nuclear receptors known as retinoic acid receptors (RARs) which are bound to DNA as heterodimers with retinoid "X" receptors (RXRs). RAR and RXR must dimerize before they can bind to the DNA. RAR will form a heterodimer with RXR (RAR-RXR), but it does not readily form a homodimer (RAR-RAR). RXR, on the other hand, may form a homodimer (RXR-RXR) and will form heterodimers with many other nuclear receptors as well, including the thyroid hormone receptor (RXR-TR), the Vitamin D_3 receptor (RXR-VDR), the peroxisome proliferator-activated receptor (RXR-PPAR) and the liver "X" receptor (RXR-LXR).

The RAR-RXR heterodimer recognizes retinoic acid response elements (RAREs) on the DNA whereas the RXR-RXR homodimer recognizes retinoid "X" response elements (RXREs) on the DNA; although several RAREs near target genes have been shown to control physiological processes, this has not been demonstrated for RXREs. The heterodimers of RXR with nuclear receptors other than RAR (i.e. TR, VDR, PPAR, LXR) bind to various distinct response elements on the DNA to control processes not regulated by vitamin A. Upon binding of retinoic acid to the RAR component of the RAR-RXR heterodimer, the receptors undergo a conformational change that causes co-repressors to dissociate from the receptors. Coactivators can then bind to the receptor complex, which may help to loosen the chromatin structure from the histones or may interact with the transcriptional machinery. This response can upregulate (or downregulate) the expression of target genes, including Hox genes as well as the genes that encode for the receptors themselves (i.e. RAR-beta in mammals).

Immune Function

Vitamin A plays a role in many areas of the immune system, particularly in T cell differentiation and proliferation.

Vitamin A promotes the proliferation of T cells through an indirect mechanism involving an increase in IL-2. In addition to promoting proliferation, Vitamin A, specifically retinoic acid, influences the differentiation of T cells. In the presence of retinoic acid, dendritic cells located in the gut are able to mediate the differentiation of T cells into regulatory T cells. Regulatory T cells are important for prevention of an immune response against "self" and regulating the strength of the immune response in order to prevent host damage. Together with TGF-β, Vitamin A promotes the conversion of T cells to regulatory T cells. Without Vitamin A, TGF-β stimulates differentiation into T cells that could create an autoimmune response.

Hematopoietic stem cells are important for the production of all blood cells, including immune cells, and are able to replenish these cells throughout the life of an individual. Dormant hematopoietic stem cells are able to self-renew and are available to differentiate and produce new blood cells when they are needed. In addition to T cells, Vitamin A is important for the correct regulation of hematopoietic stem cell dormancy. When cells are treated with all-trans retinoic acid, they are unable to leave the dormant state and become active, however, when vitamin A is removed from the diet, hematopoietic stem cells are no longer able to become dormant and the population of hematopoietic stem cells decreases. This shows an importance in creating a balanced amount of vitamin A within the environment to allow these stem cells to transition between a dormant and activated state, in order to maintain a healthy immune system.

Vitamin A has also been shown to be important for T cell homing to the intestine, effects dendritic cells, and can play a role in increased IgA secretion which is important for the immune response in mucosal tissues.

Dermatology

Vitamin A, and more specifically, retinoic acid, appears to maintain normal skin health by switching on genes and differentiating keratinocytes (immature skin cells) into mature epidermal cells. Exact mechanisms behind pharmacological retinoid therapy agents in the treatment of dermatological diseases are being researched. For the treatment of acne, the most prescribed retinoid drug is 13-cis retinoic acid (isotretinoin). It reduces the size and secretion of the sebaceous glands. Although it is known that 40 mg of isotretinoin will break down to an equivalent of 10 mg of ATRA — the mechanism of action of the drug (original brand name Accutane) remains unknown and is a matter of some controversy. Isotretinoin reduces bacterial numbers in both the ducts and skin surface. This is thought to be a result of the reduction in sebum, a nutrient source for the bacteria. Isotretinoin reduces inflammation via inhibition of chemotactic responses of monocytes and neutrophils. Isotretinoin also has been shown to initiate remodeling of the sebaceous glands; triggering changes in gene expression that selectively induce apoptosis. Isotretinoin is a teratogen with a number of potential side-effects. Consequently, its use requires medical supervision.

Retinal/Retinol versus Retinoic Acid

Vitamin A deprived rats can be kept in good general health with supplementation of retinoic acid. This reverses the growth-stunting effects of vitamin A deficiency, as well as early stages of xerophthalmia. However, such rats show infertility (in both male and females) and continued degeneration of the retina, showing that these functions require retinal or retinol, which are interconvertible but which cannot be recovered from the oxidized retinoic acid. The requirement of retinol to rescue reproduction in vitamin A deficient rats is now known to be due to a requirement for local synthesis of retinoic acid from retinol in testis and embryos.

Vitamin B

B vitamins are a class of water-soluble vitamins that play important roles in cell metabolism. Though these vitamins share similar names, they are chemically distinct compounds that often coexist in the same foods.

B vitamins are important for making sure the body's cells are functioning properly. They help the body convert food into energy (metabolism), create new blood cells, and maintain healthy skin cells, brain cells, and other body tissues.

B vitamins often occur together in the same foods. Many people can get enough B vitamins by eating a variety of nutrient-dense foods.

Vitamin B-12

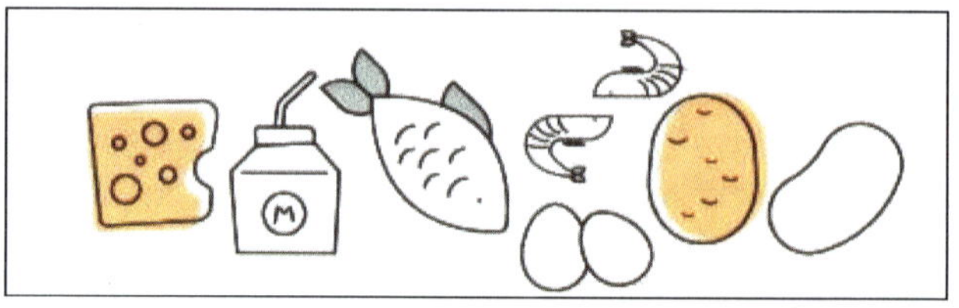

What it does: Vitamin B-12 (cobalamin) helps regulate the nervous system. It also plays a role in growth and red blood cell formation.

Which foods contain it: Vitamin B-12 is found primarily in meat and dairy products, so anyone on a strict vegan diet is at risk for deficiency. The only other dietary sources of B-12 are fortified foods.

Some of the best sources of vitamin B-12 include:

- Eggs.
- Cheese (one serving is the size of a domino).
- A glass of milk (1 cup).
- Fish (a serving of any meat is the same size as a deck of cards).
- Shellfish.
- Liver.
- Kidney.
- Red Meat.

Try this recipe for a brunch version of ratatouille. Eggs and cheese make it a great source of vitamin B-12.

What happens if you don't get enough: Vitamin B-12 deficiencies can lead to anemia and confusion in older adults.

Psychological conditions such as dementia, paranoia, depression, and behavioral changes can result from a vitamin B-12 deficiency. Neurological damage sometimes cannot be reversed.

A vitamin B-12 deficiency may cause the following symptoms:

- Tingling in the feet and hands.
- Extreme fatigue.
- Weakness.
- Irritability or depression.

Vitamin B-6

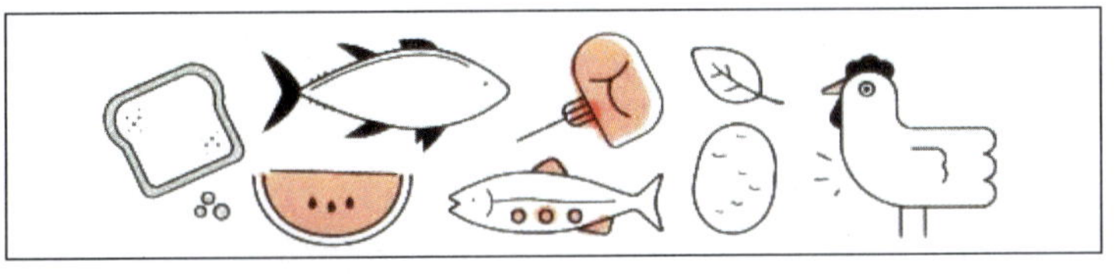

What it does: Vitamin B-6 (pyridoxine) helps the body turn food into energy. It can also help the body fight infections. Pregnant and breastfeeding women need it to help their babies' brains develop normally.

Where you get it: B-6 can be found in:

- Chickpeas.
- Tuna.
- Salmon.
- Whole grains and cereals (a portion is the size of your fist).
- Beef liver.
- Ground beef.
- Chicken breast.
- Watermelon (a serving of fruit is also no larger than a fist).
- Potatoes.
- Spinach (a serving size is equivalent to a rounded handful).

Whip up this Asian salmon and spinach rice bowl to get your daily serving of vitamin B-6.

Why you need it: Insufficient amounts of B-6 can result in anemia as well as skin disorders, such as a rash or cracks around the mouth. A lack of B-6 also can cause:

- Depression,
- Confusion,
- Nausea,
- Anemia,
- Susceptibility to infections,
- Skin rashes (dermatitis).

Vitamins B-1 and B-2

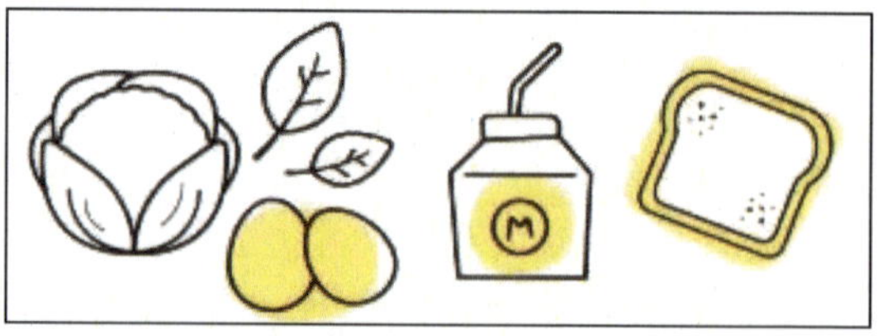

What they do: Vitamin B-1 is also called thiamin, and Vitamin B-2 is also called riboflavin. These vitamins help convert food into energy. Vitamin B-1 has neurological benefits, and vitamin B-2 helps maintain proper eyesight.

Where you get them: Most people get thiamine from breakfast cereals and whole grains. Riboflavin can be found in:

- Whole grains,
- Milk,
- Eggs,
- Dark green vegetables.

Get your daily servings of green vegetables with this green smoothie.

Why you need them: Deficiencies in thiamine and riboflavin generally don't pose a problem in the United States. This is due to the fact that many foods, such as milk and whole-grain cereals, are fortified with the vitamins. It can become an issue with people who misuse alcohol, however, presenting symptoms such as confusion and cracks along the sides of the mouth.

Vitamin B-3

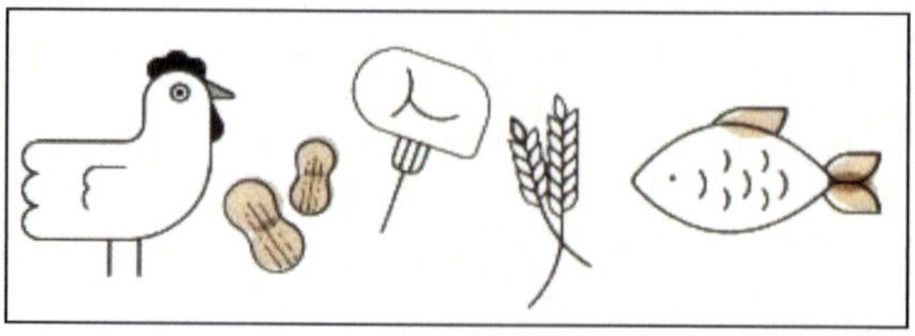

What it does: Vitamin B-3 (niacin) also helps convert food into energy. It aids in proper digestion and healthy appetite as well.

Where you get it: Niacin is found in:

- Chicken,
- Fish,
- Liver,
- Red meat,
- Whole grains, such as wheat and barley,
- Peanuts.

Why you need it: A lack of niacin can cause digestive issues, such as nausea and abdominal cramps. Severe deficiency may also cause mental confusion.

These Thai chicken tacos with peanut sauce are a great way to get niacin in your diet.

Vitamin B-9

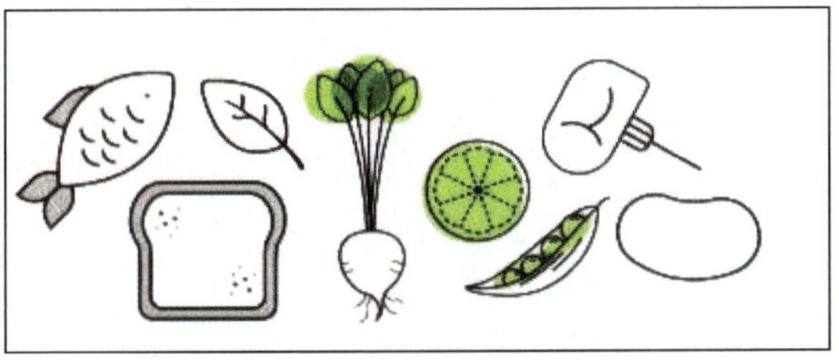

What it does: Vitamin B-9 is also called folate or folic acid. Folate is found naturally in foods. Folic acid is the synthetic form, often found in fortified, processed foods. Like most B vitamins, B-9 fosters the growth of red blood cells. It also reduces the risk of birth defects when consumed by pregnant women.

Where you get it: Vitamin B-9 can be found in:

- Meats,
- Whole grains,
- Beets,
- Citrus fruits,
- Fish,
- Fortified cereals,
- Legumes,
- Green leafy vegetables,
- Liver and kidney.

Make this spicy roasted beet hummus as a snack or appetizer.

Why you need it: Without enough folate, a person can develop diarrhea or anemia. Pregnant women with a folate deficiency could give birth to babies with defects. Excessive supplemental folic acid during pregnancy, however, may also lead to neurological problems in the baby.

Vitamin C

Vitamin C is a water-soluble vitamin. It is needed for normal growth and development.

Water-soluble vitamins dissolve in water. Leftover amounts of the vitamin leave the body through the urine. Although the body keeps a small reserve of these vitamins, they have to be taken regularly to prevent a shortage in the body.

Function

Vitamin C is needed for the growth and repair of tissues in all parts of your body. It is used to:

- Form an important protein used to make skin, tendons, ligaments, and blood vessels.
- Heal wounds and form scar tissue.
- Repair and maintain cartilage, bones and teeth.
- Aid in the absorption of iron.

Vitamin C is one of many antioxidants. Antioxidants are nutrients that block some of the damage caused by free radicals:

- Free radicals are made when your body breaks down food or when you are exposed to tobacco smoke or radiation.
- The buildup of free radicals over time is largely responsible for the aging process.
- Free radicals may play a role in cancer, heart disease, and conditions like arthritis.

The body is not able to make vitamin C on its own. It does not store vitamin C. It is therefore important to include plenty of vitamin C-containing foods in your daily diet.

Vitamin C has a definitive role in treating scurvy, which is a disease caused by vitamin C deficiency. Beyond that, a role for vitamin C as prevention or treatment for various diseases is disputed, with reviews reporting conflicting results. A Cochrane review reported no effect of vitamin C supplementation on overall mortality. It is on the World Health Organization's List of Essential Medicines as one of the most effective and safe medicines needed in a health system.

Scurvy

The disease scurvy is caused by vitamin C deficiency and can be prevented and treated with vitamin C-containing foods or dietary supplements. It takes at least a month of little to no vitamin C before symptoms occur. Early symptoms are malaise and lethargy, progressing to shortness of breath, bone pain, bleeding gums, susceptibility to bruising, poor wound healing, and finally fever, convulsions and eventual death. Until quite late in the disease the damage is reversible, as healthy collagen replaces the defective collagen with vitamin C repletion. Treatment can be orally or by intramuscular or intravenous injection. Scurvy was known to Hippocrates in the classical era. The disease was shown to be prevented by citrus fruit in an early controlled trial by a Royal Navy surgeon, James Lind, in 1747, and from 1796 lemon juice was issued to all Royal Navy crewmen.

Infection

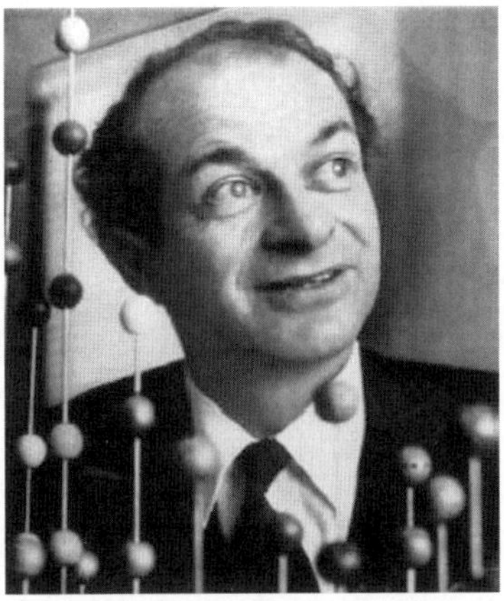

The Nobel prizewinner Linus Pauling advocated taking vitamin C for the common cold in a 1970 book.

The effect of vitamin C on the common cold has been extensively researched. The earliest publication of a controlled clinical trial appears to be from 1945. Researchers continued to work on this question, but research interest and public interest spiked after Linus Pauling, two-time awardee of the Nobel Prize, started publishing research on the topic and also published a book "Vitamin C and the Common Cold" in 1970. A revised and expanded edition "Vitamin C, the Common Cold and the Flu" was published in 1976.

Research on vitamin C in the common cold has been divided into effects on prevention, duration, and severity. A Cochrane review which looked at at least 200 mg/day concluded that vitamin C taken on a regular basis was not effective in prevention of the common cold. At least 1000 mg/day also made no difference. However, taking vitamin C on a regular basis did reduce the average duration by 8% in adults and 14% in children, and also reduced severity of colds. A subset of trials reported that supplementation reduced the incidence of colds by half in marathon runners, skiers, or soldiers in subarctic conditions. Another subset of trials looked at therapeutic use, meaning that vitamin C was not started unless the people started to feel the beginnings of a cold. In these, vitamin C did not impact duration or severity. An earlier review stated that vitamin C did not prevent colds, did reduce duration, did not reduce severity. The authors of the Cochrane review concluded that "..given the consistent effect of vitamin C on the duration and severity of colds in the regular supplementation studies, and the low cost and safety, it may be worthwhile for common cold patients to test on an individual basis whether therapeutic vitamin C is beneficial for them."

Vitamin C distributes readily in high concentrations into immune cells, has antimicrobial and natural killer cell activities, promotes lymphocyte proliferation, and is consumed quickly during infections, effects indicating a prominent role in immune system regulation. The European Food Safety Authority found a cause and effect relationship exists between the dietary intake of vitamin C and functioning of a normal immune system in adults and in children under three years of age.

Cancer

There are two approaches to the question of whether vitamin C has an impact on cancer. First, within the normal range of dietary intake without additional dietary supplementation, are people who consume more vitamin C at lower risk for developing cancer, and if so, does an orally consumed supplement have the same benefit? Second, for people diagnosed with cancer, will large amounts of ascorbic acid administered intravenously treat the cancer, reduce the adverse effects of other treatments, and so prolong survival and improve quality of life? A Cochrane review found no evidence that vitamin C supplementation reduces the risk of lung cancer in healthy people or those at high risk due to smoking or asbestos exposure. A second meta-analysis found no effect on the risk of prostate cancer. Two meta-analyses evaluated the effect of vitamin C supplementation on the risk of colorectal cancer. One found a weak association between vitamin C consumption and reduced risk, and the other found no effect from supplementation. A meta-analysis failed to find support for the prevention of breast cancer with vitamin C supplementation, but a second study concluded that vitamin C may be associated with increased survival in those already diagnosed.

Under the rubric of orthomolecular medicine, "Intravenous vitamin C is a contentious adjunctive cancer therapy, widely used in naturopathic and integrative oncology settings." With oral administration absorption efficiency decreases as amounts increase. Intravenous administration bypasses this. Doing so makes it possible to achieve plasma concentrations of 5 to 10 millimoles/liter (mmol/L), which far exceed the approximately 0.2 mmol/L limit from oral consumption. The theories of mechanism are contradictory. At high tissue concentrations ascorbic acid is described as acting as a pro-oxidant, generating hydrogen peroxide (H_2O_2) to kill tumor cells. The same literature claims that ascorbic acid acts as an antioxidant, thereby reducing the adverse effects of chemotherapy and radiation therapy. Research continues in this field, but a 2014 review concluded: "Currently, the use of high-dose intravenous vitamin C cannot be recommended outside of a clinical trial." A review added: "There is no high-quality evidence to suggest that ascorbate supplementation in cancer patients either enhances the antitumor effects of chemotherapy or reduces its toxicity. Evidence for ascorbate's anti-tumor effects was limited to case reports and observational and uncontrolled studies."

Cardiovascular Disease

A 2013 meta-analysis found no evidence that vitamin C supplementation reduces the risk of myocardial infarction, stroke, cardiovascular mortality, or all-cause mortality. However, a second analysis found an inverse relationship between circulating vitamin C levels or dietary vitamin C and the risk of stroke.

A meta-analysis of 44 clinical trials has shown a significant positive effect of vitamin C on endothelial function when taken at doses greater than 500 mg per day. The endothelium is a layer of cells that line the interior surface of blood vessels. Endothelial dysfunction is implicated in many aspects of vascular diseases. The researchers noted that the effect of vitamin C supplementation appeared to be dependent on health status, with stronger effects in those at higher risk of cardiovascular disease.

Brain Function

A 2017 systematic review found lower vitamin C concentrations in people with cognitive impairment, including Alzheimer's disease and dementia, compared to people with normal cognition. The cognitive testing, however, relied on the Mini-Mental State Examination, which is only a general test of cognition, indicating an overall low quality of research assessing the potential importance of vitamin C on cognition in normal and impaired people. A review of nutrient status in people with Alzheimer's disease reported low plasma vitamin C, but also low blood levels of folate, vitamin B_{12}, and vitamin E.

Other Diseases

Studies examining the effects of vitamin C intake on the risk of Alzheimer's disease have reached conflicting conclusions. Maintaining a healthy dietary intake is probably more important than supplementation for achieving any potential benefit. A 2010 review found no role for vitamin C supplementation in the treatment of rheumatoid arthritis. Vitamin C supplementation does not prevent or slow the progression of age-related cataract.

Side Effects

Vitamin C is a water-soluble vitamin, with dietary excesses not absorbed, and excesses in the blood rapidly excreted in the urine, so it exhibits remarkably low acute toxicity. More than two to three grams may cause indigestion, particularly when taken on an empty stomach. However, taking vitamin C in the form of sodium ascorbate and calcium ascorbate may minimize this effect. Other symptoms reported for large doses include nausea, abdominal cramps and diarrhea. These effects are attributed to the osmotic effect of unabsorbed vitamin C passing through the intestine. In theory, high vitamin C intake may cause excessive absorption of iron. A review of supplementation in healthy subjects did not report this problem but left as untested the possibility that individuals with hereditary hemochromatosis might be adversely affected.

There is a longstanding belief among the mainstream medical community that vitamin C increases risk of kidney stones. "Reports of kidney stone formation associated with excess ascorbic acid intake are limited to individuals with renal disease". Reviews state that "data from epidemiological studies do not support an association between excess ascorbic acid intake and kidney stone formation in apparently healthy individuals", although one large, multi-year trial did report a nearly two-fold increase in kidney stones in men who regularly consumed a vitamin C supplement.

Diet

Recommended Levels

US vitamin C recommendations (mg per day)	
RDA (children ages 1–3 years)	15
RDA (children ages 4–8 years)	25
RDA (children ages 9–13 years)	45
RDA (girls ages 14–18 years)	65
RDA (boys ages 14–18 years)	75
RDA (adult female)	75
RDA (adult male)	90
RDA (pregnancy)	85
RDA (lactation)	120
UL (adult female)	2,000
UL (adult male)	2,000

Recommendations for vitamin C intake by adults have been set by various national agencies:

- 40 milligrams per day: India National Institute of Nutrition, Hyderabad.
- 45 milligrams per day or 300 milligrams per week: the World Health Organization.
- 80 milligrams per day: the European Commission Council on nutrition labeling.
- 90 mg/day (males) and 75 mg/day (females): Health Canada 2007.
- 90 mg/day (males) and 75 mg/day (females): United States National Academy of Sciences.
- 100 milligrams per day: Japan National Institute of Health and Nutrition.
- 110 mg/day (males) and 95 mg/day (females): European Food Safety Authority.

In 2000 the North American Dietary Reference Intake chapter on vitamin C updated the Recommended Dietary Allowance (RDA) to 90 milligrams per day for adult men and 75 mg/day for adult women, and set a Tolerable upper intake level (UL) for adults of 2,000 mg/day. The table shows RDAs for the United States and Canada for children, and for pregnant and lactating women. For the European Union, the EFSA set higher recommendations for adults, and also for children: 20 mg/day for ages 1–3, 30 mg/day for ages 4–6, 45 mg/day for ages 7–10, 70 mg/day for ages 11–14, 100 mg/day for males ages 15–17, 90 mg/day for females ages 15–17. For pregnancy 100 mg/day; for lactation 155 mg/day. India, on the other hand, has set recommendations much lower: 40 mg/day for ages 1 through adult, 60 mg/day for pregnancy, and 80 mg/day for lactation. Clearly, there is not consensus among countries.

Cigarette smokers and people exposed to secondhand smoke have lower plasma vitamin C levels than nonsmokers. The thinking is that inhalation of smoke causes oxidative damage, depleting this antioxidant vitamin. The U.S. Institute of Medicine estimated that smokers need 35 mg more vitamin C per day than nonsmokers, but did not formally establish a higher RDA for smokers. One meta-analysis showed an inverse relationship between vitamin C intake and lung cancer, although it concluded that more research is needed to confirm this observation.

The U.S. National Center for Health Statistics conducts biannual National Health and Nutrition Examination Survey (NHANES) to assess the health and nutritional status of adults and children in the United States. Some results are reported as What We Eat In America. The 2013-2014 survey reported that for adults ages 20 years and older, men consumed on average 83.3 mg/d and women 75.1 mg/d. This means that half the women and more than half the men are not consuming the RDA for vitamin C. The same survey stated that about 30% of adults reported they consumed a vitamin C dietary supplement or a multi-vitamin/mineral supplement that included vitamin C, and that for these people total consumption was between 300 and 400 mg/d.

In 2000 the Institute of Medicine of the U.S. National Academy of Sciences set a Tolerable upper intake level (UL) for adults of 2,000 mg/day. The amount was chosen because human trials had reported diarrhea and other gastrointestinal disturbances at intakes of greater than 3,000 mg/day. This was the Lowest-Observed-Adverse-Effect Level (LOAEL), meaning that other adverse effects were observed at higher intakes. The European Food Safety Authority (EFSA) reviewed the safety question in 2006 and reached the conclusion that there was not sufficient evidence to set a UL for vitamin C. The Japan National Institute of Health and Nutrition reviewed the same question in 2010 and also reached the conclusion that there was not sufficient evidence to set a UL.

Food Labeling

For U.S. food and dietary supplement labeling purposes, the amount in a serving is expressed as a percent of Daily Value (%DV). For vitamin C labeling purposes, 100% of the Daily Value was 60 mg, but as of May 27, 2016 it was revised to 90 mg to bring it into agreement with the RDA. A table of the old and new adult Daily Values is provided at Reference Daily Intake. The original deadline to be in compliance was July 28, 2018, but on September 29, 2017 the FDA released a proposed rule that extended the deadline to January 1, 2020 for large companies and January 1, 2021 for small companies. European Union regulations require that labels declare energy, protein, fat, saturated fat, carbohydrates, sugars, and salt. Voluntary nutrients may be shown if present in significant amounts. Instead of Daily Values, amounts are shown as percent of Reference Intakes (RIs). For vitamin C, 100% RI was set at 80 mg in 2011.

The richest natural sources are fruits and vegetables. Vitamin C is the most widely taken nutritional supplement and is available in a variety of forms, including tablets, drink mixes, and in capsules.

Plant Sources

While plant foods are generally a good source of vitamin C, the amount in foods of plant origin depends on the variety of the plant, soil condition, climate where it grew, length of time since it was picked, storage conditions, and method of preparation. The following table is approximate and shows the relative abundance in different raw plant sources. As some plants were analyzed fresh while others were dried (thus, artificially increasing concentration of individual constituents like vitamin C), the data are subject to potential variation and difficulties for comparison. The amount is given in milligrams per 100 grams of the edible portion of the fruit or vegetable:

Plant source	Amount (mg/100g)
Kakadu plum	1000–5300
Camu camu	2800
Acerola	1677
Seabuckthorn	695
Indian gooseberry	445
Rose hip	426
Guava	228
Blackcurrant	200
Yellow bell pepper/capsicum	183
Red bell pepper/capsicum	128
Kale	120
Kiwifruit, broccoli	90
Green bell pepper/capsicum	80
Loganberry, redcurrant, Brussels sprouts	80
Cloudberry, elderberry	60

Papaya, strawberry	60
Orange, lemon	53
Pineapple, cauliflower	48
Cantaloupe	40
Grapefruit, raspberry	30
Passion fruit, spinach	30
Cabbage, lime	30
Mango	28
Blackberry	21
Potato, honeydew melon	20
Tomato	14
Cranberry	13
Blueberry, grape	10
Apricot, plum, watermelon	10
Avocado	8.8
Onion	7.4
Cherry, peach	7
Carrot, apple, asparagus	6

Animal Sources

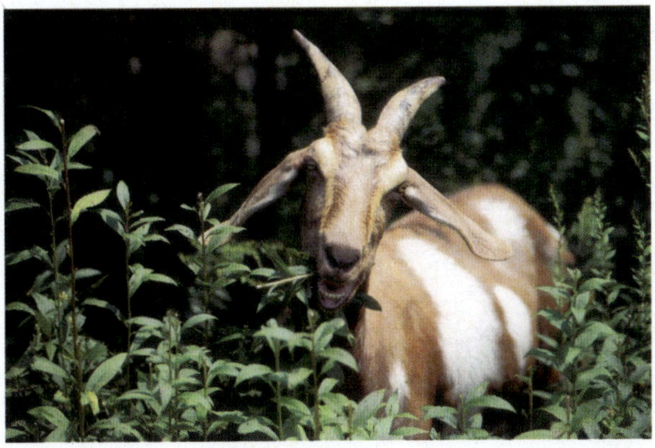

Goats, like many animals but not humans, make their own vitamin C. An adult goat, weighing approx. 70 kg, will manufacture more than 13,300 mg of vitamin C per day in normal health, and levels manyfold higher when faced with stress.

Animal-sourced foods do not provide much vitamin C, and what there is, is largely destroyed by the heat of cooking. For example, raw chicken liver contains 17.9 mg/100 g, but fried, the content is reduced to 2.7 mg/100 g. Chicken eggs contain no vitamin C, raw or cooked. Vitamin C is present in human breast milk at 5.0 mg/100 g and 6.1 mg/100 g in one tested sample of infant formula, but cow's milk contains only 1.0 mg/ 100 g.

Food Preparation

Vitamin C chemically decomposes under certain conditions, many of which may occur during the cooking of food. Vitamin C concentrations in various food substances decrease with time in proportion to the temperature at which they are stored and cooking can reduce the vitamin C content of vegetables by around 60% possibly partly due to increased enzymatic destruction as it may be more significant at sub-boiling temperatures. Longer cooking times also add to this effect, as will copper food vessels, which catalyse the decomposition.

Another cause of vitamin C being lost from food is leaching, where the water-soluble vitamin dissolves into the cooking water, which is later poured away and not consumed. However, vitamin C does not leach in all vegetables at the same rate; research shows broccoli seems to retain more than any other. Research has also shown that freshly cut fruits do not lose significant nutrients when stored in the refrigerator for a few days.

Supplements

Vitamin C dietary supplements are available as tablets, capsules, drink mix packets, in multi-vitamin/mineral formulations, in antioxidant formulations, and as crystalline powder. Vitamin C is also added to some fruit juices and juice drinks. Tablet and capsule content ranges from 25 mg to 1500 mg per serving. The most commonly used supplement compounds are ascorbic acid, sodium ascorbate and calcium ascorbate. Vitamin C molecules can also be bound to the fatty acid palmitate, creating ascorbyl palmitate, or else incorporated into liposomes.

Food Fortification

In 2014, the Canadian Food Inspection Agency evaluated the effect of fortification of foods with ascorbate in the guidance document, *Foods to Which Vitamins, Mineral Nutrients and Amino Acids May or Must be Added*. Voluntary and mandatory fortification was described for various classes of foods. Among foods classified for mandatory fortification with vitamin C were fruit-flavored drinks, mixes, and concentrates, foods for a low-energy diet, meal replacement products, and evaporated milk.

Food Additives

Ascorbic acid and some of its salts and esters are common additives added to various foods, mostly to retard oxidation. The relevant European food additive E numbers are:

1. E300 ascorbic acid (approved for use as a food additive in the EU, U.S. and Australia and New Zealand).

2. E301 sodium ascorbate (approved for use as a food additive in the EU, U.S. and Australia and New Zealand).

3. E302 calcium ascorbate (approved for use as a food additive in the EU, U.S. and Australia and New Zealand).
4. E303 potassium ascorbate (approved in Australia and New Zealand, but not in U.S.).
5. E304 fatty acid esters of ascorbic acid such as ascorbyl palmitate (approved for use as a food additive in the EU, U.S. and Australia and New Zealand).

Biosynthesis

The vast majority of animals and plants are able to synthesize vitamin C, through a sequence of enzyme-driven steps, which convert monosaccharides to vitamin C. Yeasts do not make l-ascorbic acid but rather its stereoisomer, erythorbic acid.

In plants, this is accomplished through the conversion of mannose or galactose to ascorbic acid.

In animals, the starting material is glucose. In some species that synthesize ascorbate in the liver (including mammals and perching birds), the glucose is extracted from glycogen; ascorbate synthesis is a glycogenolysis-dependent process. In animals that cannot synthesize vitamin C, the enzyme l-gulonolactone oxidase (GULO), that catalyses the last step in the biosynthesis, is highly mutated and non-functional.

Animal Pathway

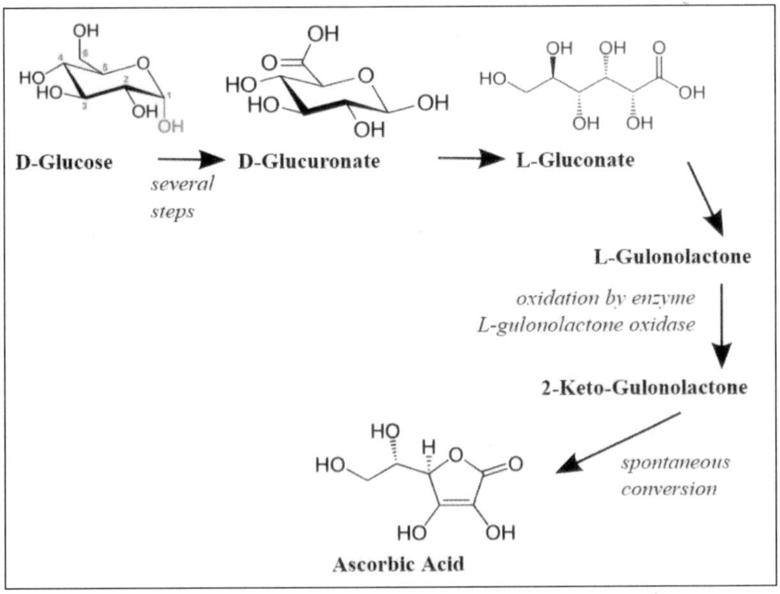

Vitamin C biosynthesis in vertebrates.

The biosynthesis of ascorbic acid in vertebrates starts with the formation of UDP-glucuronic acid. UDP-glucuronic acid is formed when UDP-glucose undergoes two oxidations catalyzed by the enzyme UDP-glucose 6-dehydrogenase. UDP-glucose 6-dehydrogenase uses the co-factor NAD^+ as the electron acceptor. The transferase UDP-glucuronate pyrophosphorylase removes a UMP and glucuronokinase, with the cofactor ADP, removes the final phosphate leading to d-glucuronic acid. The aldehyde group of this compound is reduced to a primary alcohol using the enzyme glucuronate reductase and the cofactor NADPH, yielding l-gulonic acid. This is followed by lactone formation with the hydrolase gluconolactonase between the carbonyl on C1 and hydroxyl group on C4. l-Gulonolactone then reacts with oxygen, catalyzed by the enzyme l-gulonolactone oxidase (which is nonfunctional in humans and other Haplorrhini primates) and the cofactor FAD^+. This reaction produces 2-oxogulonolactone (2-keto-gulonolactone), which spontaneously undergoes enolization to form ascorbic acid.

Some mammals have lost the ability to synthesize vitamin C, including simians and tarsiers, which together make up one of two major primate suborders, Haplorrhini. This group includes humans. The other more primitive primates (Strepsirrhini) have the ability to make vitamin C. Synthesis does not occur in most bats nor in species in the rodent family Caviidae, that includes guinea pigs and capybaras, but does occur in other rodents, including rats and mice.

Reptiles and older orders of birds make ascorbic acid in their kidneys. Recent orders of birds and most mammals make ascorbic acid in their liver. A number of species of passerine birds also do not synthesize, but not all of them, and those that do not are not clearly related; there is a theory that the ability was lost separately a number of times in birds. In particular, the ability to synthesize vitamin C is presumed to have been lost and then later re-acquired in at least two cases. The ability to synthesize vitamin C has also been lost in about 96% of fish (the teleosts).

Most tested families of bats (order Chiroptera), including major insect and fruit-eating bat families, cannot synthesize vitamin C. A trace of gulonolactone oxidase was detected in only 1 of 34 bat species tested, across the range of 6 families of bats tested. There are at least two species of bats, frugivorous bat (*Rousettus leschenaultii*) and insectivorous bat (*Hipposideros armiger*), that retain (or regained) their ability of vitamin C production.

Some of these species (including humans) are able to make do with the lower levels available from their diets by recycling oxidised vitamin C.

Most simians consume the vitamin in amounts 10 to 20 times higher than that recommended by governments for humans. This discrepancy constitutes much of the basis of the controversy on current recommended dietary allowances. It is countered by arguments that humans are very good at conserving dietary vitamin C, and are able to maintain blood levels of vitamin C comparable with simians on a far smaller dietary intake, perhaps by recycling oxidized vitamin C.

Plant Pathways

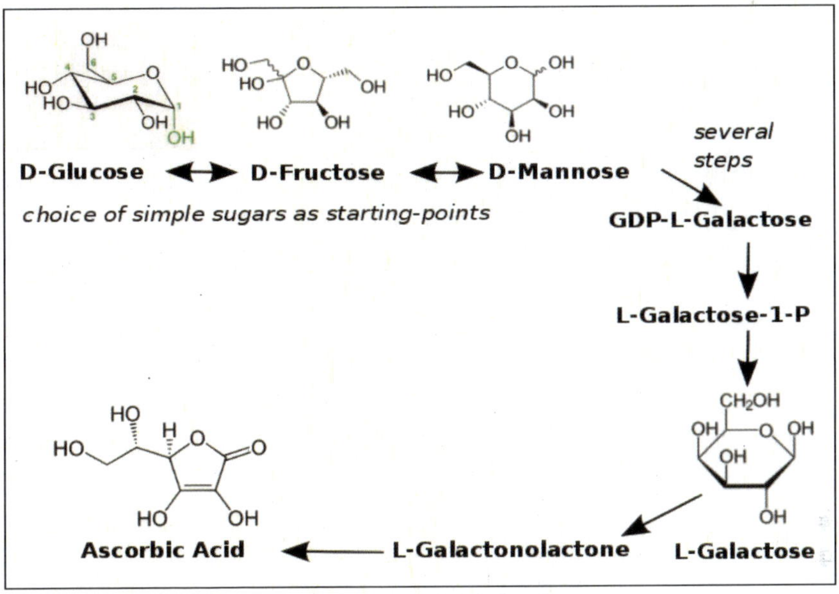

Vitamin C biosynthesis in plants.

There are many different biosynthesis pathways for ascorbic acid in plants. Most of these pathways are derived from products found in glycolysis and other pathways. For example, one pathway goes through the plant cell wall polymers. The plant ascorbic acid biosynthesis pathway most principal seems to be L-galactose. L-Galactose reacts with the enzyme L-galactose dehydrogenase, whereby the lactone ring opens and forms again but with between the carbonyl on C1 and hydroxyl group on the C4, resulting in L-galactonolactone. L-Galactonolactone then reacts with the mitochondrial flavoenzyme L-galactonolactone dehydrogenase. to produce ascorbic acid. L-Ascorbic acid has a negative feedback on L-galactose dehydrogenase in spinach. Ascorbic acid efflux by embryo of dicots plants is a well-established mechanism of iron reduction, and a step obligatory for iron uptake.

All plants synthesize ascorbic acid. Ascorbic acid functions as a cofactor for enzymes involved in photosynthesis, synthesis of plant hormones, as an antioxidant and also regenerator of other antioxidants. Plants use multiple pathways to synthesize vitamin C. The major pathway starts with glucose, fructose or mannose (all simple sugars) and proceeds to L-galactose, L-galactonolactone and ascorbic acid. There is feedback regulation in place, in that the presence of ascorbic acid inhibits enzymes in the synthesis pathway. This process follows a diurnal rhythm, so that enzyme expression peaks in the morning to support biosynthesis later on when mid-day sunlight intensity demands high ascorbic acid concentrations. Minor pathways may be specific to certain parts of plants; these can be either identical to the vertebrate pathway (including the GLO enzyme), or start with inositol and get to ascorbic acid via L-galactonic acid to L-galactonolactone.

Evolution

Ascorbic acid is a common enzymatic cofactor in mammals used in the synthesis of collagen, as well as a powerful reducing agent capable of rapidly scavenging a number of reactive oxygen species (ROS). Given that ascorbate has these important functions, it is surprising that the ability to synthesize this molecule has not always been conserved. In fact, anthropoid primates, *Cavia porcellus* (guinea pigs), teleost fishes, most bats, and some Passeriform birds have all independently lost the ability to internally synthesize Vitamin C in either the kidney or the liver. In all of the cases where genomic analysis was done on an ascorbic acid auxotroph, the origin of the change was found to be a result of loss-of-function mutations in the gene that codes for L-Gulono-γ-lactone oxidase, the enzyme that catalyzes the last step of the ascorbic acid pathway outlined above. One explanation for the repeated loss of the ability to synthesize vitamin C is that it was the result of genetic drift; assuming that the diet was rich in vitamin C, natural selection would not act to preserve it.

In the case of the simians, it is thought that the loss of the ability to make vitamin C may have occurred much farther back in evolutionary history than the emergence of humans or even apes, since it evidently occurred soon after the appearance of the first primates, yet sometime after the split of early primates into the two major suborders Haplorrhini (which cannot make vitamin C) and its sister suborder of non-tarsier prosimians, the Strepsirrhini ("wet-nosed" primates), which retained the ability to make vitamin C. According to molecular clock dating, these two suborder primate branches parted ways about 63 to 60 million years ago. Approximately three to five million years later (58 million years ago), only a short time afterward from an evolutionary perspective, the infraorder Tarsiiformes, whose only remaining family is that of the tarsier (Tarsiidae), branched off from the other haplorrhines. Since tarsiers also cannot make vitamin C, this implies the mutation had already occurred, and thus must have occurred between these two marker points (63 to 58 million years ago).

It has also been noted that the loss of the ability to synthesize ascorbate strikingly parallels the inability to break down uric acid, also a characteristic of primates. Uric acid and ascorbate are both strong reducing agents. This has led to the suggestion that, in higher primates, uric acid has taken over some of the functions of ascorbate.

Vitamin D

Vitamin D is a group of fat-soluble secosteroids responsible for increasing intestinal absorption of calcium, magnesium, and phosphate, and multiple other biological effects. In humans, the most important compounds in this group are vitamin D_3 (also known as cholecalciferol) and vitamin D_2 (ergocalciferol).

The major natural source of the vitamin is synthesis of cholecalciferol in the skin from cholesterol through a chemical reaction that is dependent on sun exposure (specifically UVB radiation). Cholecalciferol and ergocalciferol can be ingested from the diet and from supplements. Only a few foods, such as the flesh of fatty fish, contain significant amounts of vitamin D, and fish does not contain enough vitamin D to achieve optimal Vitamin D status without sunlight or supplements. Dietary recommendations typically assume that all of a person's vitamin D is taken by mouth, as sun exposure in the population is variable and recommendations about the amount of sun exposure that is safe are uncertain in view of the skin cancer risk.

Vitamin D from the diet, or from skin synthesis, is biologically inactive. A protein enzyme must hydroxylate it to convert it to the active form. This is done in the liver and in the kidneys. As vitamin D can be synthesized in adequate amounts by most mammals exposed to sufficient sunlight, it is not an essential dietary factor, and so not technically a vitamin. Instead it could be considered a hormone, with activation of the vitamin D pro-hormone resulting in the active form, calcitriol, which then produces effects via a nuclear receptor in multiple locations.

Cholecalciferol is converted in the liver to calcifediol (25-hydroxycholecalciferol); ergocalciferol is converted to 25-hydroxyergocalciferol. These two vitamin D metabolites (called 25-hydroxyvitamin D or 25(OH)D) are measured in serum to determine a person's vitamin D status. Calcifediol is further hydroxylated by the kidneys to form calcitriol (also known as 1,25-dihydroxycholecalciferol), the biologically active form of vitamin D. Calcitriol circulates as a hormone in the blood, having a major role regulating the concentration of calcium and phosphate, and promoting the healthy growth and remodeling of bone. Calcitriol also has other effects, including some on cell growth, neuromuscular and immune functions, and reduction of inflammation.

Vitamin D has a significant role in calcium homeostasis and metabolism. Its discovery was due to effort to find the dietary substance lacking in children with rickets (the childhood form of osteomalacia). Vitamin D supplements are given to treat or to prevent osteomalacia and rickets, but the evidence for other health effects of vitamin D supplementation in the general population is inconsistent. The effect of vitamin D supplementation on mortality is not clear, with one meta-analysis finding a small decrease in mortality in elderly people, and another concluding no clear justification exists for recommending supplementation for preventing many diseases, and that further research of similar design is unneeded in these areas.

Types

Name	Chemical composition	Structure
Vitamin D_1	Mixture of molecular compounds of ergocalciferol with lumisterol, 1:1.	
Vitamin D_2	Ergocalciferol (made from ergosterol).	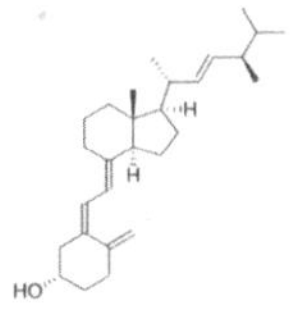

Vitamin D_3	Cholecalciferol (made from 7-dehydrocholesterol in the skin).	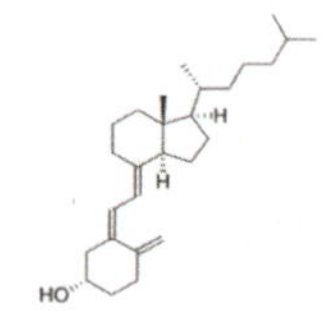
Vitamin D_4	22-dihydroergocalciferol.	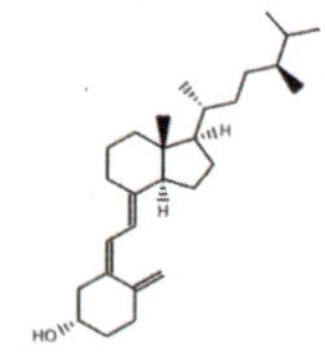
Vitamin D_5	Sitocalciferol (made from 7-dehydrositosterol).	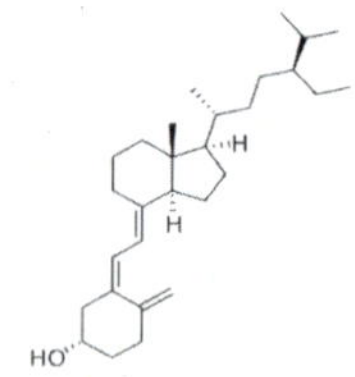

Several forms (vitamers) of vitamin D exist. The two major forms are vitamin D_2 or ergocalciferol, and vitamin D_3 or cholecalciferol; vitamin D without a subscript refers to either D_2 or D_3 or both. These are known collectively as calciferol. Vitamin D_2 was chemically characterized in 1931. In 1935, the chemical structure of vitamin D_3 was established and proven to result from the ultraviolet irradiation of 7-dehydrocholesterol.

Chemically, the various forms of vitamin D are secosteroids, i.e., steroids in which one of the bonds in the steroid rings is broken. The structural difference between vitamin D_2 and vitamin D_3 is the side chain of D_2 contains a double bond between carbons 22 and 23, and a methyl group on carbon 24.

Biology

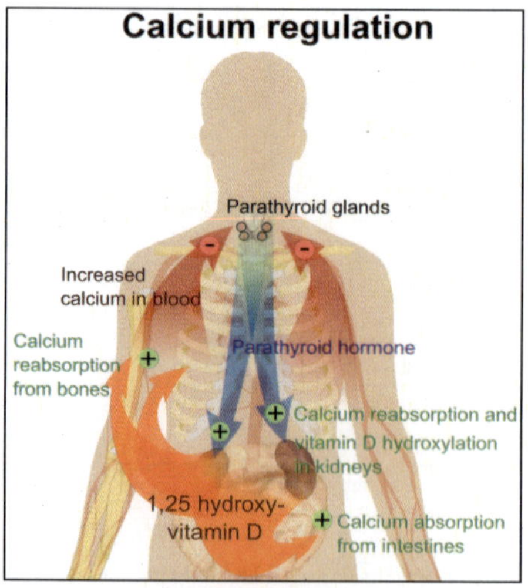

Calcium regulation in the human body. The role of active vitamin D (1,25-dihydroxyvitamin D, calcitriol) is shown in orange.

The active vitamin D metabolite calcitriol mediates its biological effects by binding to the vitamin D receptor (VDR), which is principally located in the nuclei of target cells. The binding of calcitriol to the VDR allows the VDR to act as a transcription factor that modulates the gene expression of transport proteins (such as TRPV6 and calbindin), which are involved in calcium absorption in the intestine. The vitamin D receptor belongs to the nuclear receptor superfamily of steroid/thyroid hormone receptors, and VDRs are expressed by cells in most organs, including the brain, heart, skin, gonads, prostate, and breast.

VDR activation in the intestine, bone, kidney, and parathyroid gland cells leads to the maintenance of calcium and phosphorus levels in the blood (with the assistance of parathyroid hormone and calcitonin) and to the maintenance of bone content.

One of the most important roles of vitamin D is to maintain skeletal calcium balance by promoting calcium absorption in the intestines, promoting bone resorption by increasing osteoclast number, maintaining calcium and phosphate levels for bone formation, and allowing proper functioning of parathyroid hormone to maintain serum calcium levels. Vitamin D deficiency can result in lower bone mineral density and an increased risk of reduced bone density (osteoporosis) or bone fracture because a lack of vitamin D alters mineral metabolism in the body. Thus, vitamin D is also critical for bone remodeling through its role as a potent stimulator of bone resorption.

The VDR regulates cell proliferation and differentiation. Vitamin D also affects the immune system, and VDRs are expressed in several white blood cells, including monocytes and activated T and B cells. In vitro, vitamin D increases expression of the tyrosine hydroxylase gene in adrenal medullary cells, and affects the synthesis of neurotrophic factors, nitric oxide synthase, and glutathione.

Deficiency

A diet with insufficient vitamin D in conjunction with inadequate sun exposure causes vitamin D deficiency. Severe vitamin D deficiency in children causes rickets, a softening and weakening of bones, which is a rare disease in the developed world. Vitamin D deficiency is found worldwide in the elderly and remains common in children and adults. Deficiency results in impaired bone mineralization and bone damage which leads to bone-softening diseases, including rickets in children and osteomalacia in adults. Low blood calcifediol (25-hydroxy-vitamin D) can result from avoiding the sun. Being deficient in vitamin D can cause intestinal absorption of dietary calcium to fall to 15%. When not deficient, an individual usually absorbs between 60-80%.

Bone Health

Rickets

Rickets, a childhood disease, is characterized by impeded growth and soft, weak, deformed long bones that bend and bow under their weight as children start to walk. This condition is characterized by bow legs, which can be caused by calcium or phosphorus deficiency, as well as a lack of vitamin D; today, it is largely found in low-income countries in Africa, Asia, or the Middle East and in those with genetic disorders such as pseudovitamin D deficiency rickets.

Maternal vitamin D deficiency may cause overt bone disease from before birth and impairment of bone quality after birth. Nutritional rickets exists in countries with intense year-round sunlight such as Nigeria and can occur without vitamin D deficiency.

Although rickets and osteomalacia are now rare in the UK, outbreaks have happened in some immigrant communities in which osteomalacia sufferers included women with seemingly adequate daylight outdoor exposure wearing Western clothing. Having darker skin and reduced exposure to sunshine did not produce rickets unless the diet deviated from a Western omnivore pattern characterized by high intakes of meat, fish, and eggs, and low intakes of high-extraction cereals. The dietary risk factors for rickets include abstaining from animal foods.

Vitamin D deficiency remains the main cause of rickets among young infants in most countries, because breast milk is low in vitamin D and social customs and climatic conditions can prevent adequate sun exposure. In sunny countries such as Nigeria, South Africa, and Bangladesh, where rickets occurs among older toddlers and children, it has been attributed to low dietary calcium intakes, which are characteristic of cereal-based diets with limited access to dairy products.

Rickets was formerly a major public health problem among the US population; in Denver, where ultraviolet rays are about 20% stronger than at sea level on the same latitude, almost two-thirds of 500 children had mild rickets in the late 1920s. An increase in the proportion of animal protein in the 20th century American diet coupled with increased consumption of milk fortified with relatively small quantities of vitamin D coincided with a dramatic decline in the number of rickets cases. Also, in the United States and Canada, vitamin D-fortified milk, infant vitamin supplements, and vitamin supplements have helped to eradicate the majority of cases of rickets for children with fat malabsorption conditions.

Osteoporosis and Osteomalacia

Osteomalacia is a disease in adults that results from vitamin D deficiency. Characteristics of this disease are softening of the bones, leading to bending of the spine, bowing of the legs, proximal muscle weakness, bone fragility, and increased risk for fractures. Osteomalacia reduces calcium absorption and increases calcium loss from bone, which increases the risk for bone fractures. Osteomalacia is usually present when 25-hydroxyvitamin D levels are less than about 10 ng/mL. Although the effects of osteomalacia are thought to contribute to chronic musculoskeletal pain, there is no persuasive evidence of lower vitamin D levels in chronic pain sufferers or that supplementation alleviates chronic nonspecific musculoskeletal pain.

Skin Pigmentation

Dark-skinned people living in temperate climates have been shown to have low vitamin D levels but the significance of this is not certain. Dark-skinned people are less efficient at making vitamin D because melanin in the skin hinders vitamin D synthesis.

Uses of Supplements

The effects of vitamin D supplementation on health are uncertain. A 2013 review did not find any effect from supplementation on the rates of disease, other than a tentative decrease in mortality in the elderly. Vitamin D supplements do not alter the outcomes for myocardial infarction, stroke or cerebrovascular disease, cancer, bone fractures or knee osteoarthritis. Low vitamin D levels may result from disease rather than cause disease.

A United States Institute of Medicine report states: "Outcomes related to cancer, cardiovascular disease and hypertension, and diabetes and metabolic syndrome, falls and physical performance, immune functioning and autoimmune disorders, infections, neuropsychological functioning, and preeclampsia could not be linked reliably with calcium or vitamin D intake and were often conflicting." Some researchers claim the IOM was too definitive in its recommendations and made a mathematical mistake when calculating the blood level of vitamin D associated with bone health. Members of the IOM panel maintain that they used a "standard procedure for dietary recommendations" and that the report is solidly based on the data. Research on vitamin D supplements, including large-scale clinical trials, is continuing.

Mortality

Vitamin D_3 supplementation has been tentatively found to lead to a reduced risk of death in the elderly, but the effect has not been deemed pronounced, or certain enough, to make taking supplements recommendable. Other forms (vitamin D_2, alfacalcidol, and calcitriol) do not appear to have any beneficial effects with regard to the risk of death. High blood levels appear to be associated with a lower risk of death, but it is unclear if supplementation can result in this benefit. Both an excess and a deficiency in vitamin D appear to cause abnormal functioning and premature aging. The relationship between serum calcifediol level and all-cause mortality is parabolic. Harm from vitamin D appears to occur at a lower vitamin D level in the black population than in the white population.

Bone Health

In general, no good evidence supports the commonly held belief that vitamin D supplements can help prevent osteoporosis. Its general use for prevention of this disease in those without vitamin D deficiency is thus likely not needed. For older people with osteoporosis, taking vitamin D with calcium may help prevent hip fractures, but it also slightly increases the risk of stomach and kidney problems. Supplementation with higher doses of vitamin D, in those older than 65 years, may decrease fracture risk. The effect is small or none for people living independently. Low serum vitamin D levels have been associated with falls, and low bone mineral density. Taking extra vitamin D, however, does not appear to change the risk. Athletes who are vitamin D deficient are at an increased risk of stress fractures and/or major breaks, particularly those engaging in contact sports. The greatest benefit with supplementation is seen in athletes who are deficient (25(OH)D serum levels <30 ng/mL), or severely deficient (25(OH)D serum levels <25 ng/mL). Incremental decreases in risks are observed with rising serum 25(OH)D concentrations plateauing at 50 ng/mL with no additional benefits seen in levels beyond this point.

Because it found mounting evidence for a benefit to bone health, though it had not found good evidence of other benefits, the US Food and Drug Administration (FDA) has required manufacturers to declare the amount of vitamin D on nutrition facts labels, as "nutrients of public health significance", since May 2016. By a proposed deadline extension, small manufacturers with less than $10 million in annual food sales will have to comply by January 1, 2021, while larger ones have to comply by January 1, 2020. Manufacturers of single-ingredient sugars such as honey and maple syrup and certain cranberry products have until July 1, 2021, to make the changes.

Cancer

Vitamin D supplements have been widely marketed for their claimed anticancer properties. Associations have been shown in observational studies between low vitamin D levels and the risk of development of certain cancers. It is unclear, however, if taking additional vitamin D in the diet or as supplements affects the risk of cancer. Reviews have described the evidence as being "inconsistent, inconclusive as to causality, and insufficient to inform nutritional requirements" and "not sufficiently robust to draw conclusions". One 2014 review found that supplements had no significant effect on cancer risk.

Another 2014 review concluded that vitamin D_3 may decrease the risk of death from cancer (one fewer death in 150 people treated over 5 years), but concerns with the quality of the data were noted. Insufficient evidence exists to recommend vitamin D supplements for people with cancer, although some evidence suggests that low vitamin D may be associated with a worse outcome for some cancers, and that higher 25-hydroxy vitamin D levels at the time of diagnosis are associated with better outcomes.

Cardiovascular Disease

Taking vitamin D supplements does not meaningfully reduce the risk of stroke, cerebrovascular disease, cardial infarction, or ischemic heart disease. Supplementation may have no effect on blood pressure.

Immune System

Infectious Diseases

In general, vitamin D functions to activate the innate and dampen the adaptive immune systems. Deficiency has been linked to increased risk or severity of viral infections, including HIV. Low levels of vitamin D appear to be a risk factor for tuberculosis, and historically it was used as a treatment. Supplementation slightly decreases the risk of acute respiratory tract infections and the exacerbation of asthma. Evidence is lacking on whether it does so in children under five years of age. No clinical trials have been done to assess its effect on preventing other infections, such as malaria.

Autoimmune Diseases

Although tentative data link low levels of vitamin D to asthma, evidence to support a beneficial effect on asthmatics from supplementation is inconclusive. Accordingly, supplementation is not currently recommended for treatment or prevention of asthma. Vitamin D and multiple sclerosis incidence have been linked, but it is not clear what the nature of any causal relationship might be. Two systemic reviews concluded that the evidence for vitamin D supplementation being helpful for treating people with multiple sclerosis is inconclusive.

Inflammatory Bowel Disease

Low levels of vitamin D are associated with two major forms of human Inflammatory bowel disease (IBD): Crohn's disease and ulcerative colitis. However, further studies are required to determine its significance and the potential role of vitamin D axis in IBD.

Other Conditions

1. Diabetes: A systematic review of 2014 concluded that the available studies show no evidence of vitamin D3 supplementation having an effect on glucose homeostasis or diabetes prevention. Vitamin D deficiency may be a risk factor for diabetes, over-all evidence regarding vitamin D levels and diabetes mellitus is contradictory, requiring further studies.

2. Depression: Clinical trials of vitamin D supplementation for depressive symptoms have generally been of low quality and show no overall effect, although subgroup analysis showed supplementation for participants with clinically significant depressive symptoms or depressive disorder had a moderate effect.

3. Cognition and dementia: A systematic review of clinical studies found an association between low vitamin D levels with cognitive impairment and a higher risk of developing Alzheimer's disease: However, lower vitamin D concentrations are also associated with poor nutrition and spending less time outdoors.

Therefore, alternative explanations for the increase in cognitive impairment exist and hence a direct causal relationship between vitamin D levels and cognition could not be established.

4. Pregnancy: Low levels of vitamin D in pregnancy are associated with gestational diabetes, pre-eclampsia, and small (for gestational age) infants. Although taking vitamin D supplements during pregnancy raises blood levels of vitamin D in the mother at term, the extent of benefits for the mother or baby is unclear. Pregnant women who take an adequate amount of vitamin D during gestation may experience a lower risk of pre-eclampsia and positive immune effects. A 2018 review found that supplements may reduce the risk of undersized babies and of their poor rate of growth. Pregnant women often do not take the recommended amount of vitamin D.
5. Weight loss: Though hypothesized that vitamin D supplementation may be an effective treatment for obesity apart from calorie restriction, one systematic review found no association of supplementation with body weight or fat mass. A 2016 meta-analysis found that circulating vitamin D status was improved by weight loss, indicating that fat mass may be inversely associated with blood levels of vitamin D.

Allowable Health Claims

Governmental regulatory agencies stipulate for the food and dietary supplement industries certain health claims as allowable as statements on packaging.

1. European Food Safety Authority.
    - Normal function of the immune system.
    - Normal inflammatory response.
    - Normal muscle function.
    - Reduced risk of falling in people over age 60.
2. US Food and Drug Administration (FDA).
    - "Adequate calcium and vitamin D, as part of a well balanced diet, along with physical activity, may reduce the risk of osteoporosis".
3. Health Canada.
    - Adequate calcium and regular exercise may help to achieve strong bones in children and adolescents and may reduce the risk of osteoporosis in older adults. An adequate intake of vitamin D is also necessary.

Other possible agencies with claim guidance: Japan FOSHU and Australia-New Zealand.

Dietary Intake

Recommended Levels

United States		
Age group	RDA (IU/day)	(μg/day)
Infants 0–6 months	400*	10
Infants 6–12 months	400*	10
1–70 years	600	15
71+ years	800	20
Pregnant/Lactating	600	15
Age group	Tolerable upper intake level (IU/day)	(μg/day)
Infants 0–6 months	1,000	25
Infants 6–12 months	1,500	37.5
1–3 years	2,500	62.5
4–8 years	3,000	75
9+ years	4,000	100
Pregnant/lactating	4,000	100
Canada		
Age group	RDA (IU)	Tolerable upper intake (IU)
Infants 0–6 months	400*	1,000
Infants 7–12 months	400*	1,500
Children 1–3 years	600	2,500
Children 4–8 years	600	3,000
Children and Adults 9–70 years	600	4,000
Adults > 70 years	800	4,000
Pregnancy & Lactation	600	4,000
Australia and New Zealand		
Age group	Adequate Intake (μg)	Upper Level of Intake (μg)
Infants 0–12 months	5*	25
Children 1–18 years	5*	80
Adults 19–50 years	5*	80
Adults 51–70 years	10*	80
Adults > 70 years	15*	80
European Food Safety Authority		
Age group	Adequate Intake (μg)	Tolerable upper limit (μg)
Infants 0–12 months	10	25
Children 1–10 years	15	50
Children 11–17 years	15	100
Adults	15	100
Pregnancy & Lactation	15	100
* Adequate intake, no RDA/RDI yet established		

Conversion: 1 μg = 40 IU.

Various institutions have proposed different recommendations for the amount of daily intake of vitamin D. These vary according to precise definition, age, pregnancy or lactation, and the extent assumptions are made regarding skin synthesis of vitamin D.

United States

The dietary reference intake for vitamin D issued in 2010 by the Institute of Medicine (IoM) (renamed National Academy of Medicine in 2015), superseded previous recommendations which were expressed in terms of Adequate Intake. The recommendations were formed assuming the individual has no skin synthesis of vitamin D because of inadequate sun exposure. The reference intake for vitamin D refers to total intake from food, beverages and supplements, and assumes that calcium requirements are being met. The tolerable upper intake level (UL) is defined as "the highest average daily intake of a nutrient that is likely to pose no risk of adverse health effects for nearly all persons in the general population." Although ULs are believed to be safe, information on the long-term effects is incomplete and these levels of intake are not recommended for long-term consumption.

For U.S food and dietary supplement labeling purposes, the amount in a serving is expressed as a percent of Daily Value (%DV). For vitamin D labeling purposes, 100% of the Daily Value was 400 IU (10 μg), but on May 27, 2016, it was revised to 800 IU (20 μg) to bring it into agreement with the RDA. The deadline to be in compliance was extended to January 1, 2020 for large companies and January 1, 2021 for small companies.

Canada

Health Canada published recommended dietary allowances (RDA) and tolerable upper intake levels for vitamin D in 2012 based on the Institute of Medicine report.

Australia and New Zealand

Australia and New Zealand published nutrient reference values including guidelines for dietary vitamin D intake in 2005. About a third of Australians have vitamin D deficiency.

European Union

The European Food Safety Authority (EFSA) in 2016 reviewed the current evidence, finding the relationship between serum 25(OH)D concentration and musculoskeletal health outcomes is widely variable. They considered that average requirements and population reference intakes values for vitamin D cannot be derived, and that a serum 25(OH)D concentration of 50 nmol/L was a suitable target value. For all people over the age of 1, including women who are pregnant or lactating, they set an adequate intake of 15 μg/day (600 IU).

The EFSA reviewed safe levels of intake in 2012, setting the tolerable upper limit for adults at 100 µg/day (4000 IU), a similar conclusion as the IOM.

The UK National Health Service recommends babies and young children aged six months to five years, pregnant or breastfeeding women, and sun-deprived elderly people should take daily vitamin supplements to ensure sufficient vitamin D intake. In July 2016, Public Health England recommended that everyone consider taking a daily supplement containing 10 µg of vitamin D during autumn and winter because of inadequate sunlight for vitamin D synthesis.

The Swedish National Food Agency recommends a daily intake of 10 µg (400 IU) of vitamin D3 for children and adults up to 75 years, and 20 µg (800 IU) for adults 75 and older.

Non-government organisations in Europe have made their own recommendations. The German Society for Nutrition recommends 20 µg. The European Menopause and Andropause Society recommends postmenopausal women consume15 µg (600 IU) until age 70, and 20 µg (800 IU) from age 71. This dose should be increased to 100 µg (4,000 IU) in some patients with very low vitamin D status or in case of co-morbid conditions.

Although vitamin D is not present naturally in most foods, it is commonly added as a fortification in manufactured foods. In some countries, staple foods are artificially fortified with vitamin D.

Natural Sources

In general, vitamin D_2 is found in fungi and vitamin D_3 is found in animals. Vitamin D_2 is produced by ultraviolet irradiation of ergosterol found in many fungi. The vitamin D_2 content in mushrooms and *Cladina arbuscula*, a lichen, increase with exposure to ultraviolet light. This process is emulated by industrial ultraviolet lamps, concentrating vitamin D_2 levels to higher levels.

The United States Department of Agriculture reports D_2 and D_3 content combined in one value.

Fungal sources			
Source		µg/g	IU/g
C. arbuscula (lichen), thalli, dry	vitamin D_3	0.67–2.04	27–82
	vitamin D_2	0.22–0.55	8.8–22
Agaricus bisporus (common mushroom): $D_2 + D_3$			
Portobello	Raw	0.003	0.1
	Exposed to ultraviolet light	0.112	4.46
Crimini	Raw	0.001	0.03
	Exposed to ultraviolet light	0.319	12.76

Animal sources		
Source	IU/g	Irregular
Cooked egg yolk	0.7	44 IU for a 61g egg
Beef liver, cooked, braised	0.5	
Fish liver oils, such as cod liver oil	100	450 IU per teaspoon (4.5 g)
Fatty fish species		
Salmon, pink, cooked, dry heat	5.2	
Mackerel, Pacific and jack, mixed species, cooked, dry heat	4.6	
Tuna, canned in oil	2.7	
Sardines, canned in oil, drained	1.9	

Food Fortification

Manufactured foods fortified with vitamin D include some fruit juices and fruit juice drinks, meal replacement energy bars, soy protein-based beverages, certain cheese and cheese products, flour products, infant formulas, many breakfast cereals, and milk.

In 2016 in the United States, the Food and Drug Administration (FDA) amended food additive regulations for milk fortification, stating that vitamin D_3 levels not exceed 42 IU vitamin D per 100 g (400 IU per US quart) of dairy milk, 84 IU of vitamin D_2 per 100 g (800 IU per quart) of plant milks, and 89 IU per 100 g (800 IU per quart) in plant-based yogurts or in soy beverage products. Plant milks are defined as beverages made from soy, almond, rice, among other plant sources intended as alternatives to dairy milk.

While some studies have found that vitamin D_3 raises 25(OH)D blood levels faster and remains active in the body longer, others contend that vitamin D_2 sources are equally bioavailable and effective as D_3 for raising and sustaining 25(OH)D.

Food Preparation

Vitamin D content in typical foods is reduced variably by cooking. Boiled, fried and baked foods retained 69–89% of original vitamin D.

Biosynthesis

Synthesis of vitamin D in nature is dependent on the presence of UV radiation and subsequent activation in liver and in kidney. Many animals synthesize vitamin D_3 from 7-dehydrocholesterol, and many fungi synthesize vitamin D_2 from ergosterol.

Photochemistry

The transformation that converts 7-dehydrocholesterol to vitamin D_3 occurs in two steps. First, 7-dehydrocholesterol is photolyzed by ultraviolet light in a 6-electron conrotatory ring-opening electrocyclic reaction; the product is previtamin D_3. Second, previtamin D_3 spontaneously isomerizes to vitamin D_3 (cholecalciferol) in an antarafacial sigmatropic hydride shift. At room temperature, the transformation of previtamin D_3 to vitamin D_3 in an organic solvent takes about 12 days to complete. The conversion of previtamin D_3 to vitamin D_3 in the skin is about 10 times faster than in an organic solvent.

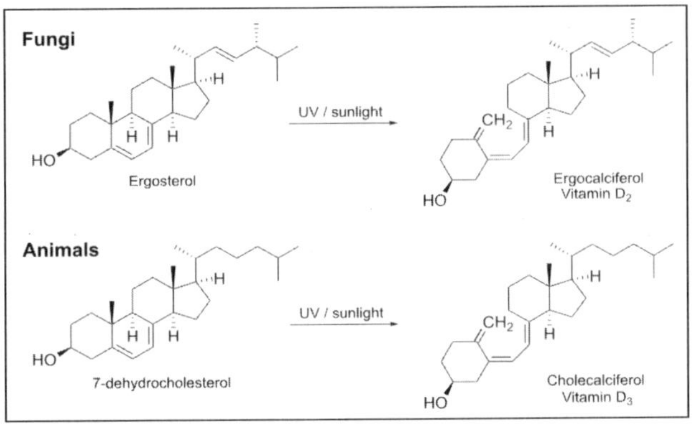

The photochemistry of vitamin D biosynthesis in animal and fungi.

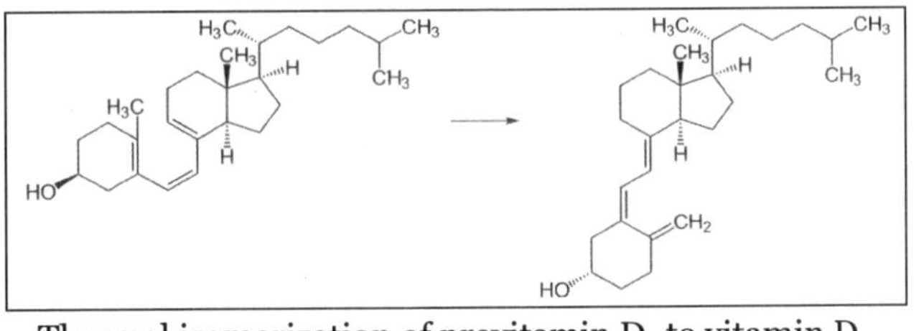

Thermal isomerization of previtamin D_3 to vitamin D_3.

The conversion from ergosterol to vitamin D_2 follows a similar procedure, forming previtamin D_2 by photolysis, which isomerizes to vitamin D_2. The transformation of previtamin D_2 to vitamin D_2 in methanol has a rate comparable to that of previtamin D_3. The process is faster in white button mushrooms.

Synthesis in the Skin

Vitamin D_3 is produced photochemically from 7-dehydrocholesterol in the skin of most vertebrate animals, including humans. The precursor of vitamin D_3, 7-dehydrocholesterol is produced in relatively large quantities. 7-Dehydrocholesterol reacts with UVB light at wavelengths of 290–315 nm. These wavelengths are present in sunlight, as well as in the light emitted by the UV lamps in tanning beds (which produce ultraviolet primarily in the UVA spectrum, but typically produce 4% to 10% of the total UV emissions as UVB). Exposure to light through windows is insufficient because glass almost completely blocks UVB light.

Adequate amounts of vitamin D can be produced with moderate sun exposure to the face, arms and legs, averaging 5–30 minutes twice per week, or approximately 25%

of the time for minimal sunburn. The darker the skin, and the weaker the sunlight, the more minutes of exposure are needed. Vitamin D overdose is impossible from UV exposure; the skin reaches an equilibrium where the vitamin degrades as fast as it is created.

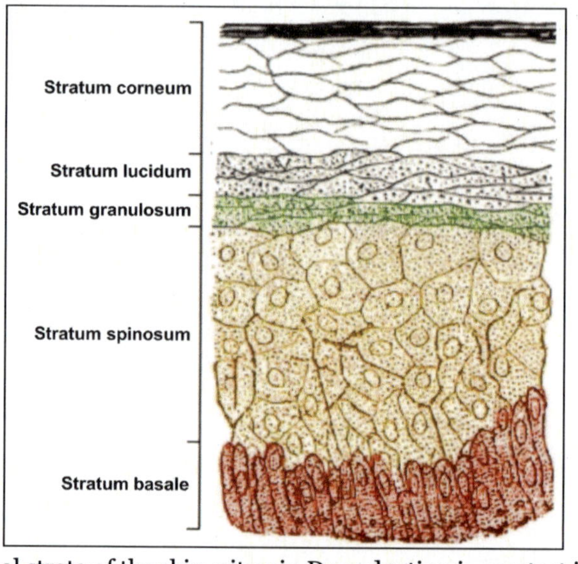

In the epidermal strata of the skin, vitamin D production is greatest in the stratum basale (colored red in the illustration) and stratum spinosum (colored light brown).

Sunscreen absorbs or reflects ultraviolet light and prevents much of it from reaching the skin. Sunscreen with a sun protection factor (SPF) of 8 based on the UVB spectrum decreases vitamin D synthetic capacity by 95%, and SPF 15 decreases it by 98%.

The skin consists of two primary layers: the inner layer called the dermis, composed largely of connective tissue, and the outer, thinner epidermis. Thick epidermis in the soles and palms consists of five strata; from outer to inner, they are: the stratum corneum, stratum lucidum, stratum granulosum, stratum spinosum, and stratum basale. Vitamin D is produced in the keratinocytes of two innermost strata, the stratum basale and stratum spinosum.

Evolution

Vitamin D can be synthesized only by a photochemical process. Phytoplankton in the ocean (such as coccolithophore and *Emiliania huxleyi*) have been photosynthesizing vitamin D for more than 500 million years. Primitive vertebrates in the ocean could absorb calcium from the ocean into their skeletons and eat plankton rich in vitamin D.

Land vertebrates required another source of vitamin D other than plants for their calcified skeletons. They had to either ingest it or be exposed to sunlight to photosynthesize it in their skin. Land vertebrates have been photosynthesizing vitamin D for more than 350 million years.

In birds and fur-bearing mammals, fur or feathers block UV rays from reaching the skin. Instead, vitamin D is created from oily secretions of the skin deposited onto the feathers or fur, and is obtained orally during grooming. However, some animals, such as the naked mole-rat, are naturally cholecalciferol-deficient, as serum 25-OH vitamin D levels are undetectable.

Industrial Synthesis

Vitamin D_3 (cholecalciferol) is produced industrially by exposing 7-dehydrocholesterol to UVB light, followed by purification. The 7-dehydrocholesterol is a natural substance in fish organs, especially the liver, or in wool grease (lanolin) from sheep. Vitamin D_2 (ergocalciferol) is produced in a similar way using ergosterol from yeast or mushrooms as a starting material.

Mechanism of Action

Metabolic Activation

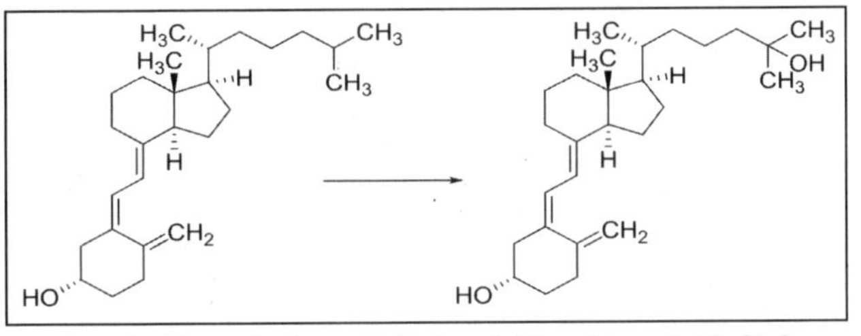

Liver hydroxylation of cholecalciferol to calcifediol.

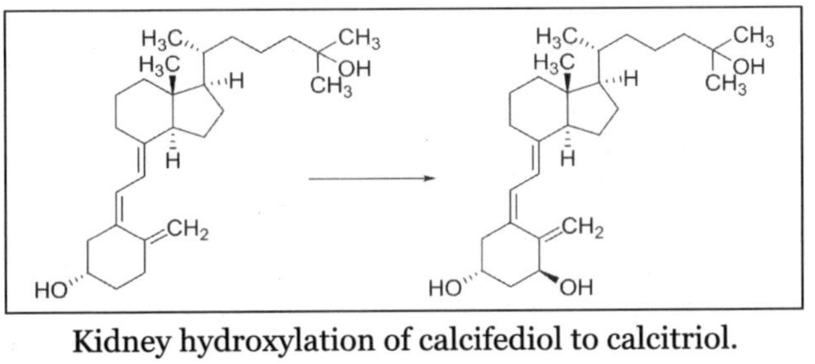

Kidney hydroxylation of calcifediol to calcitriol.

Vitamin D is carried in the bloodstream to the liver, where it is converted into the prohormone calcifediol. Circulating calcifediol may then be converted into calcitriol, the biologically active form of vitamin D, in the kidneys.

Whether it is made in the skin or ingested, vitamin D is hydroxylated in the liver at position 25 (upper right of the molecule) to form 25-hydroxycholecalciferol (calcifediol or 25(OH)D). This reaction is catalyzed by the microsomal enzyme vitamin D 25-hydroxylase, the product of the *CYP2R1* human gene, and expressed by hepatocytes. Once made, the product is released into the plasma, where it is bound to an α-globulin carrier protein named the vitamin D-binding protein.

Calcifediol is transported to the proximal tubules of the kidneys, where it is hydroxylated at the 1-α position (lower right of the molecule) to form calcitriol (1,25-dihydroxycholecalciferol, 1,25(OH)$_2$D). The conversion of calcifediol to calcitriol is catalyzed by the enzyme 25-hydroxyvitamin D$_3$ 1-alpha-hydroxylase, which is the product of the *CYP27B1* human gene. The activity of CYP27B1 is increased by parathyroid hormone, and also by low calcium or phosphate.

Following the final converting step in the kidney, calcitriol is released into the circulation. By binding to vitamin D-binding protein, calcitriol is transported throughout the body, including to the classical target organs of intestine, kidney and bone. Calcitriol is the most potent natural ligand of the vitamin D receptor, which mediates most of the physiological actions of vitamin D.

In addition to the kidneys, calcitriol is also synthesized by certain other cells including monocyte-macrophages in the immune system. When synthesized by monocyte-macrophages, calcitriol acts locally as a cytokine, modulating body defenses against microbial invaders by stimulating the innate immune system.

Inactivation

The activity of calcifediol and calcitriol can be reduced by hydroxylation at position 24 by vitamin D$_3$ 24-hydroxylase, forming secalciferol and calcitetrol, respectively.

Difference between Substrates

Vitamin D$_2$ (ergocalciferol) and vitamin D$_3$ (cholecaliferol) share a similar mechanism of action as outlined above. Metabolites produced by vitamin D$_2$ are sometimes named with an *er-* or *ergo* prefix to differentiate them from the D$_3$-based counterparts.

- Metabolites produced from vitamin D$_2$ tend to bind less well to the vitamin D-binding protein.
- Vitamin D$_3$ can alternatively be hydroxylated to calcifediol by sterol 27-hydroxylase (CYP27A1), but vitamin D$_2$ cannot.
- Ergocalciferol can be directly hydroxylated at position 24. This hydroxylation also leads to a greater degree of inactivation: while calcitriol's activity decreases to 60% of original after 24-hydroxylation, ercalcitriol suffers a 10-fold decrease in activity on conversion to ercalcitetrol.

Vitamin E

Vitamin E is a group of eight fat soluble compounds that include four tocopherols and four tocotrienols. Vitamin E deficiency, which is rare and usually due to an underlying problem with digesting dietary fat rather than from a diet low in vitamin E, can cause nerve problems. Vitamin E is a fat-soluble antioxidant protecting cell membranes from reactive oxygen species.

Worldwide, government organizations recommend adults consume in the range of 7 to 15 mg per day. As of 2016, consumption was below recommendations according to a worldwide summary of more than one hundred studies that reported a median dietary intake of 6.2 mg per day for alpha-tocopherol. Research with alpha-tocopherol as a dietary supplement, with daily amounts as high as 2000 mg per day, has had mixed results. Population studies suggested that people who consumed foods with more vitamin E, or who chose on their own to consume a vitamin E dietary supplement, had lower incidence of cardiovascular diseases, cancer, dementia, and other diseases, but placebo-controlled clinical trials could not always replicate these findings, and there were some indications that vitamin E supplementation actually was associated with a modest increase in all-cause mortality. As of 2017, vitamin E continues to be a topic of active clinical research. There is no clinical evidence that use of vitamin E skincare products are effective.

Both the tocopherols and tocotrienols occur in α (alpha), β (beta), γ (gamma) and δ (delta) forms, as determined by the number and position of methyl groups on the chromanol ring. All eight of these vitamers feature a chromane double ring, with a hydroxyl group that can donate a hydrogen atom to reduce free radicals, and a hydrophobic side chain which allows for penetration into biological membranes. Of the many different forms of vitamin E, gamma-tocopherol (γ-tocopherol) is the most common form found in the North American diet, but alpha-tocopherol (α-tocopherol) is the most biologically active. Palm oil is a source of tocotrienols.

Vitamin E was discovered in 1922, isolated in 1935 and first synthesized in 1938. Because the vitamin activity was first identified as essential for fertilized eggs to result in live births (in rats), it was given the name "tocopherol" from Greek words meaning *birth* and *to bear* or *carry*. Alpha-tocopherol, either naturally extracted from plant oils or synthetic, is sold as a popular dietary supplement, either by itself or incorporated into a multivitamin product, and in oils or lotions for use on skin.

Functions

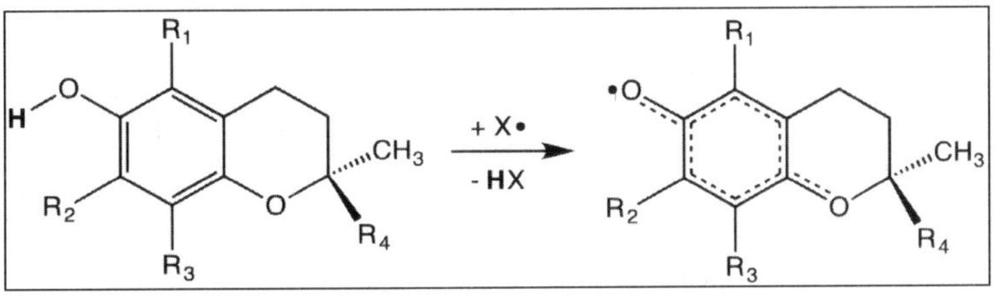

Tocopherols function by donating H atoms to radicals (X).

Vitamin E may have various roles as a vitamin. Many biological functions have been postulated, including a role as a fat-soluble antioxidant. In this role, vitamin E acts as a radical scavenger, delivering a hydrogen (H) atom to free radicals. At 323 kJ/mol, the O-H bond in tocopherols is about 10% weaker than in most other phenols. This weak bond allows the vitamin to donate a hydrogen atom to the peroxyl radical and other free radicals, minimizing their damaging effect. The thus-generated tocopheryl radical is recycled to tocopherol by a redox reaction with a hydrogen donor, such as vitamin C. As it is fat-soluble, vitamin E is incorporated into cell membranes, which are therefore protected from oxidative damage.

Vitamin E affects gene expression and is an enzyme activity regulator, such as for protein kinase C (PKC) – which plays a role in smooth muscle growth – with vitamin E participating in deactivation of PKC to inhibit smooth muscle growth.

Deficiency

Vitamin E deficiency is rare in humans, occurring as a consequence of abnormalities in dietary fat absorption or metabolism rather than from a diet low in vitamin E. One example of a genetic abnormality in metabolism is mutations of genes coding for alpha-tocopherol transfer protein (α-TTP). Humans with this genetic defect exhibit a progressive neurodegenerative disorder known as ataxia with vitamin E deficiency (AVED) despite consuming normal amounts of vitamin E. Large amounts of alpha-tocopherol as a dietary supplement are needed to compensate for the lack of α-TTP Vitamin E deficiency due to either malabsorption or metabolic anomaly can cause nerve problems due to poor conduction of electrical impulses along nerves due to changes in nerve membrane structure and function. In addition to ataxia, vitamin E deficiency can cause peripheral neuropathy, myopathies, retinopathy and impairment of immune responses.

Side Effects

The U.S. Food and Nutrition Board set a Tolerable upper intake level (UL) at 1,000 mg (1,500 IU) per day derived from animal models that demonstrated bleeding at high doses. The European Food Safety Authority reviewed the same safety question and set a UL at 300 mg/day. A meta-analysis of long-term clinical trials reported a non-significant 2% increase in all-cause mortality when alpha-tocopherol was the only supplement used. The same meta-analysis reported a statistically significant 3% increase for results when alpha-tocopherol was used by itself or in combination with other nutrients (vitamin A, vitamin C, beta-carotene, selenium). Another meta-analysis reported a non-significant 1% increase in all-cause mortality when alpha-tocopherol was the only supplement. Subset analysis reported no difference between natural (plant extracted) or synthetic alpha-tocopherol, or whether the amount used was less than or more than 400 IU/day. There are reports of vitamin E-induced allergic contact dermatitis from use of vitamin-E derivatives such as tocopheryl linoleate and tocopherol acetate in skin care products. Incidence is low despite widespread use.

Drug Interactions

The amounts of alpha-tocopherol, other tocopherols and tocotrienols that are components of dietary vitamin E, when consumed from foods, do not appear to cause any interactions with drugs. Consumption of alpha-tocopherol as a dietary supplement in amounts in excess of 300 mg/day may lead to interactions with aspirin, warfarin, tamoxifen and cyclosporine A in ways that alter function. For aspirin and warfarin, high amounts of vitamin E may potentiate anti-blood clotting action. One small trial demonstrated that vitamin E at 400 mg/day reduced blood concentration of the anti-breast cancer drug tamoxifen. In multiple clinical trials, vitamin E lowered blood concentration of the immunosuppressant medication, cyclosporine A. The US National Institutes of Health, Office of Dietary Supplements, raises a concern that co-administration of vitamin E could counter the mechanisms of anti-cancer radiation therapy and some types of chemotherapy, and so advises against its use in these patient populations. The references it cited reported instances of reduced treatment adverse effects, but also poorer cancer survival, raising the possibility of tumor protection from the intended oxidative damage by the treatments.

Diet

Recommendations

US vitamin E recommendations (mg per day)	
AI (children ages 0–6 months)	4
AI (children ages 7–12 months)	5
RDA (children ages 1–3 years)	6
RDA (children ages 4–8 years)	7
RDA (children ages 9–13 years)	11
RDA (children ages 14–18 years)	15
RDA (adults ages 19+)	15
RDA (pregnancy)	15
RDA (lactation)	19
UL (adults)	1,000

The U.S. Institute of Medicine (renamed National Academy of Medicine in 2015) updated Estimated Average Requirements (EARs) and Recommended Dietary Allowances (RDAs) for vitamin E in 2000. The EAR for vitamin E for women and men ages 14 and up is 12 mg/day. The RDA is 15 mg/day. RDAs are higher than EARs so as to identify amounts that will cover people with higher than average requirements. For infants up to 12 months the Adequate Intake (AI) is 4–5 mg/day. As for safety, Tolerable upper intake levels (ULs) are set for vitamins and minerals when evidence is sufficient. Hemorrhagic effects in rats were selected as the critical endpoint to calculate the UL via starting with the lowest-observed-adverse-effect-level (LOAEL) and processing that through an uncertainty factor calculation. The end result was a UL set at 1000 mg/day. Collectively the EARs, RDAs, AIs and ULs are referred to as Dietary Reference Intakes (DRIs).

The European Food Safety Authority (EFSA) refers to the collective set of information as Dietary Reference Values, with Population Reference Intake (PRI) instead of RDA, and Average Requirement instead of EAR. AI and UL defined the same as in United States. For women and men ages 10 and older the PRIs are set at 11 and 13 mg/day, respectively. PRI for pregnancy is 11 mg/day, for lactation 11 mg/day. For children ages 1–9 years the PRIs increase with age from 6 to 9 mg/day. These PRIs are lower than the U.S. RDAs. The European Food Safety Authority reviewed the same safety question and set a UL at 300 mg/day. The EU used an effect on blood clotting as a critical effect, identified that no adverse effects were observed in a human trial as 540 mg/day, used an uncertainty factor of 2 to get to a suggest UL of 270 mg/day, then rounded up to 300 mg/day.

The Japan National Institute of Health and Nutrition set lower AIs than the U.S. RDAs or EU PRIs, and intermediate ULs: 6.5 mg/day (females) and 7.0 mg/day (males) for adult AIs, and 650–700 mg/day (females) and 750–900 mg/day (males) for adult ULs, amount depending on age. India recommends an intake of 8–10 mg/day and does not set a UL. The World Health Organization recommends that adults consume 10 mg/day.

Consumption is below government recommendations. A worldwide summary of more than one hundred studies reported a median dietary intake of 6.2 mg/d for alpha-tocopherol. Government survey results in the U.S. reported average consumption for adult females at 8.4 mg/d and adult males 10.4 mg/d. Both are both below the RDA of 15 mg/day.

Food Labeling

For U.S. food and dietary supplement labeling purposes the amount in a serving is expressed as a percent of Daily Value (%DV). For vitamin E labeling purposes 100% of the Daily Value was 30 IU, but as of May 27, 2016 it was revised to 15 mg to bring it into agreement with the RDA. A table of the old and new adult Daily Values is provided at Reference Daily Intake. The original deadline to be in compliance was July 28, 2018, but on September 29, 2017 the FDA released a proposed rule that extended the deadline to January 1, 2020 for large companies and January 1, 2021 for small companies. European Union regulations require that labels declare energy, protein, fat, saturated fat, carbohydrates, sugars, and salt. Voluntary nutrients may be shown if present in significant amounts. Instead of Daily Values, amounts are shown as percent of Reference Intakes (RIs). For vitamin E, 100% RI was set at 12 mg in 2011.

The U.S. Department of Agriculture (USDA), Agricultural Research Services, maintains a food composition database. The last major revision was Release 28, September 2015. In addition to the naturally occurring sources shown in the table, certain ready-to-eat cereals, infant formulas, liquid nutrition products and other foods are fortified with alpha-tocopherol.

Plant source	Amount (mg/100g)
Wheat germ oil	150
Hazelnut oil	47
Canola/rapeseed oil	44
Sunflower oil	41.1
Safflower oil	34.1
Almond oil	39.2
Grapeseed oil	28.8
Sunflower seed kernels	26.1
Almonds	25.6
Almond butter	24.2
Wheat germ	19
Canola oil	17.5
Palm oil	15.9
Peanut oil	15.7
Margarine, tub	15.4
Hazelnuts	15.3
Corn oil	14.8
Olive oil	14.3
Soybean oil	12.1
Pine nuts	9.3
Peanut butter	9.0
Peanuts	8.3
Popcorn	5.0
Pistachio nuts	2.8
Mayonnaise	3.3
Avocados	2.6
Spinach, raw	2.0
Asparagus	1.5
Broccoli	1.4
Cashew nuts	0.9
Bread	0.2-0.3
Rice, brown	0.2
Potato, Pasta	<0.1
Fish	1.0-2.8
Oysters	1.7
Butter	1.6
Cheese	0.6-0.7
Eggs	1.1
Chicken	0.3
Beef	0.1
Pork	0.1
Milk, whole	0.1
Milk, skim	0.01

Supplements

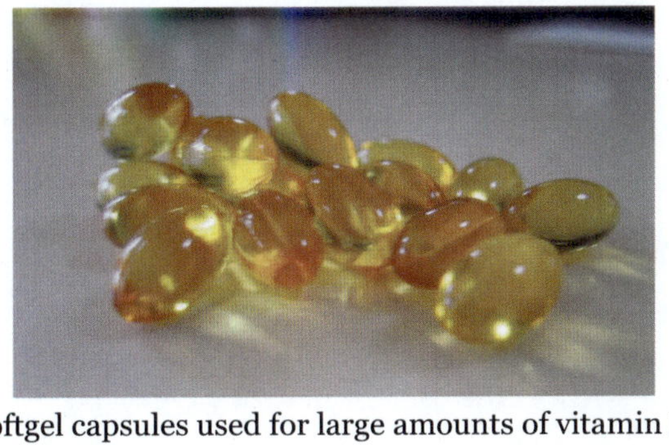

Softgel capsules used for large amounts of vitamin E.

Vitamin E is fat soluble, so dietary supplement products are usually in the form of the vitamin dissolved in vegetable oil in a softgel capsule. For alpha-tocopherol, amounts range from 100 to 1000 IU per serving. Smaller amounts are incorporated into multi-vitamin/mineral tablets. Gamma-tocopherol and tocotrienol supplements are also available from dietary supplement companies. The latter are extracts from palm or annatto oils.

Fortification

The World Health Organization does not have any recommendations for food fortification with vitamin E. The Food Fortification Initiative does not list any countries that have mandatory or voluntary programs for vitamin E. Infant formulas have alpha-tocopherol as an ingredient. In some countries, certain brands of ready-to-eat cereals, liquid nutrition products and other foods have alpha-tocopherol as an added ingredient.

Metabolism

Tocotrienols and tocopherols, the latter including the stereoisomers of synthetic alpha-tocopherol, are absorbed from the intestinal lumen, incorporated into chylomicrons, and secreted into the portal vein, leading to the liver. Absorption efficiency is estimated at 51% to 86%, and that applies to all of the vitamin E family–there is no discrimination among the vitamin E vitamers during absorption. Unabsorbed vitamin E is excreted via feces. Additionally, vitamin E is excreted by the liver via bile into the intestinal lumin, where it will either be reabsorbed or excreted via feces, and all of the vitamin E vitamers are metabolized and then excreted via urine.

Upon reaching the liver, RRR-alpha-tocopherol is preferentially taken up by alpha-tocopherol transfer protein (α-TTP). All other forms are degraded to 2'-carboxethyl-6-hydroxychromane (CEHC), a process that involves truncating the phytic tail of the molecule, then either sulfated or glycuronidated. This renders the molecules water-soluble and leads to excretion via urine. Alpha-tocopherol is also degraded by the same process, to 2,5,7,8-tetramethyl-2-(2'-carboxyethyl)-6-hydroxychromane (α-CEHC), but more slowly because it is partially protected by α-TTP. Large intakes of α-tocopherol result in increased urinary α-CEHC, so this appears to be a means of disposing of excess vitamin E.

Alpha-tocopherol transfer protein is coded by the TTPA gene on chromosome 8. The binding site for RRR-α-tocopherol is a hydrophobic pocket with a lower affinity for beta-, gamma-, or delta-tocopherols, or for the stereoisomers with an S configuration at the chiral 2 site. Tocotrienols are also a poor fit because the double bonds in the phytic tail create a rigid configuration that is a mismatch with the α-TTP pocket. A rare genetic defect of the TTPA gene results in people exhibiting a progressive neurodegenerative disorder known as ataxia with vitamin E deficiency (AVED) despite consuming normal amounts of vitamin E. Large amounts of alpha-tocopherol as a dietary supplement are needed to compensate for the lack of α-TTP The role of α-TTP is to move α-tocopherol to the plasma membrane of hepatocytes (liver cells), where in can be incorporated into newly created very low density lipoprotein (VLDL) molecules. These convey α-tocopherol to cells in the rest of the body. As an example of a result of the preferential treatment, the US diet delivers approximately 70 mg/d of γ-tocopherol and plasma concentrations are on the order of 2–5 μmol/L; meanwhile. dietary α-tocopherol is about 7 mg/d but plasma concentrations are in the range of 11–37 μmol/L.

Affinity of α-TTP for Vitamin E Vitamers

Vitamin E Compound	Affinity
RRR-alpha-tocopherol	100%
Beta-tocopherol	38%
Gamma-tocopherol	9%
Delta-tocopherol	2%
SSR-alpha-tocopherol	11%
Alpha-tocotrienol	12%

Synthesis

Biosynthesis

Photosynthesizing plants, algae and cyanobacteria synthesize tocochromanols, the chemical family of compounds made up of four tocopherols and four tocotrienols; in a nutrition context this family is referred to as Vitamin E. Biosynthesis starts with formation of the closed-ring part of the molecule as homogentisic acid (HGA). The side chain is attached (saturated for tocopherols, polyunsaturated for tocotrienols). The pathway for both is the same, so that gamma- is created and from that alpha-, or delta- is created and from that the beta- compounds. Biosynthesis takes place in the plastids.

As to why plants synthesize tocochromanols, the major reason appears to be for antioxidant activity. Different parts of plants, and different species, are dominated by different tocochromamols. The predominant form in leaves, and hence leafy green vegetables is α-tocopherol. Location is in chloroplast membranes, this in close proximity to the photosynthetic process. The function is to protect against damage from the ultraviolet radiation of sunlight. Under normal growing conditions the presence of α-tocopherol does not appear to be essential, as there are other photo-protective compounds, and plant mutations that have lost the ability to synthesize α-tocopherol demonstrate normal growth. However, under stressed growing conditions such as drought, elevated temperature or salt-induced oxidative stress, the plants' physiological status is superior if it has the normal synthesis capacity.

Seeds are lipid-rich, to provide energy for germination and early growth. Tocochromanols protect the seed lipids from oxidizing and becoming rancid. The presence of tocochromanols extends seed longevity, and promotes successful germination and seedling growth. Gamma-tocopherol dominates in seeds of most plant species, but there are exceptions. For canola, corn and soy bean oils, there is more γ-tocopherol than α-tocopherol, but for safflower, sunflower and olive oils the reverse is true. Of the commonly used food oils, palm oil is unique in that tocotrienol content is higher than tocopherol content. Seed tocochromanols content is also dependent on environmental stressors. In almonds, for example, drought or elevated temperature increase α-tocopherol and γ-tocopherol content of the nuts. The same topic mentions that drought increases the tocopherol content of olives, and heat likewise for soybeans.

Industrial Synthesis

Naturally sourced d-alpha-tocopherol can be extracted and purified from seed oils, or gamma-tocopherol can be extracted, purified, and methylated to create d-alpha-tocopherol. In contrast to alpha-tocopherol extracted from plants, which is also called d-alpha-tocopherol, industrial synthesis creates dl-alpha-tocopherol. "It is synthesized from a mixture of toluene and 2,3,5-trimethyl-hydroquinone that reacts with isophytol to all-rac-alpha-tocopherol, using iron in the presence of hydrogen chloride gas as catalyst. The reaction mixture obtained is filtered and extracted with aqueous caustic soda. Toluene is removed by evaporation and the residue (all rac-alpha-tocopherol) is purified by vacuum distillation." Specification for the ingredient is >97% pure. This synthetic dl-alpha-tocopherol has approximately 50% of the potency of d-alpha-tocopherol. Manufacturers of dietary supplements and fortified foods for humans or domesticated animals convert the phenol form of the vitamin to an ester using either acetic acid or succinic acid because the esters are more chemically stable, providing for a longer shelf-life. The ester forms are de-esterified in the gut and absorbed as free alpha-tocopherol.

Vitamin K

Vitamin K is a group of structurally similar, fat-soluble vitamins found in foods and in dietary supplements. The human body requires vitamin K for complete synthesis of certain proteins that are needed for blood coagulation (K from *Koagulation*, German for "coagulation") or for controlling binding of calcium in bones and other tissues. The vitamin K-related modification of the proteins allows them to bind calcium ions, which they cannot do otherwise. Without vitamin K, blood coagulation is seriously impaired, and uncontrolled bleeding occurs. Preliminary clinical research indicates that deficiency of vitamin K may weaken bones, potentially leading to osteoporosis, and may promote calcification of arteries and other soft tissues.

Chemically, the vitamin K family comprises 2-methyl-1,4-naphthoquinone (3-) derivatives. Vitamin K includes two natural vitamers: vitamin K_1 and vitamin K_2. Vitamin K_2, in turn, consists of a number of related chemical subtypes, with differing lengths of carbon side chains made of isoprenoid groups of atoms.

Vitamin K_1, also known as phylloquinone, is made by plants, and is found in highest amounts in green leafy vegetables because it is directly involved in photosynthesis. It may be thought of as the plant form of vitamin K. It is active as a vitamin in animals and performs the classic functions of vitamin K, including its activity in the production of blood-clotting proteins. Animals may also convert it to vitamin K_2.

Bacteria in the gut flora can also convert K_1 into vitamin K_2 (menaquinone). In addition, bacteria typically lengthen the isoprenoid side chain of vitamin K_2 to produce a range of vitamin K_2 forms, most notably the MK-7 to MK-11 homologues of vitamin K_2. All forms of K_2 other than MK-4 can only be produced by bacteria, which use these during anaerobic respiration. The MK-7 and other bacterially derived forms of vitamin K_2 exhibit vitamin K activity in animals, but MK-7's extra utility over MK-4, if any, is unclear and is a matter of investigation.

Because a synthetic form of vitamin K, vitamin K_3 (menadione), may be toxic by interfering with the function of glutathione, it is no longer used to treat vitamin K deficiency.

Medical Uses

Warfarin Overdose and Coumarin Poisoning

Vitamin K is one of the treatments for bleeding events caused by overdose of the anticoagulant drug warfarin (Coumadin®). It can be administered by mouth, intravenously, or subcutaneously. Vitamin K is also used in situations when a patient's INR is greater than 10 and there is no active bleeding.

Vitamin K is also part of the suggested treatment regime for poisoning by rodenticide (coumarin poisoning). Vitamin K treatment may only be necessary in people who deliberately have consumed large amounts of rodenticide or have consumed an unknown amount of rodenticide. Patients should be given oral Vitamin K_1 to prevent the negative effects of rodenticide poisoning. Oral Vitamin K_1 is preferred over other routes of administration because it has less side effects.

Vitamin K Deficiency Bleeding in Newborns

Vitamin K is given as an injection to newborns to prevent Vitamin K deficiency bleeding. The blood clotting factors of newborn babies are roughly 30–60% that of adult values; this may be due to the reduced synthesis of precursor proteins and the sterility of their guts. Human milk contains 1–4 μg/L of vitamin K_1, while formula-derived milk can contain up to 100 μg/L in supplemented formulas. Vitamin K_2 concentrations in human milk appear to be much lower than those of vitamin K_1. Occurrence of vitamin K deficiency bleeding in the first week of the infant's life is estimated at 0.25–1.7%, with a prevalence of 2–10 cases per 100,000 births. Premature babies have even lower levels of the vitamin, so they are at a higher risk from this deficiency.

Bleeding in infants due to vitamin K deficiency can be severe, leading to hospitalization, blood transfusions, brain damage, and death. Supplementation can prevent most cases of vitamin K deficiency bleeding in the newborn. Intramuscular administration (known as the *Vitamin K shot*) is more effective in preventing late vitamin K deficiency bleeding than oral administration.

Osteoporosis

There is no good evidence that vitamin K supplementation benefits the bone health of postmenopausal women.

Cardiovascular Health

Adequate intake of vitamin K is associated with the inhibition of arterial calcification and stiffening, but there have been few interventional studies and no good evidence that vitamin K supplementation is of any benefit in the primary prevention of cardiovascular disease.

One 10-year population study, the Rotterdam Study, did show a clear and significant inverse relationship between the highest intake levels of menaquinone (mainly MK-4 from eggs and meat, and MK-8 and MK-9 from cheese) and cardiovascular disease and all-cause mortality in older men and women.

Cancer

Vitamin K has been promoted in supplement form with claims it can slow tumor growth; however, no good medical evidence supports such claims.

Side Effects

Although allergic reaction from supplementation is possible, no known toxicity is associated with high doses of the phylloquinone (vitamin K_1) or menaquinone (vitamin K_2) forms of vitamin K, so no tolerable upper intake level (UL) has been set. Specifically vitamin K_1 has been associated with severe adverse reactions such as bronchospasm and cardiac arrest when given intravenously as opposed to orally.

Blood clotting (coagulation) studies in humans using 45 mg per day of vitamin K_2 (as MK-4) and even up to 135 mg per day (45 mg three times daily) of K_2 (as MK-4), showed no increase in blood clot risk. Even doses in rats as high as 250 mg/kg, body weight did not alter the tendency for blood-clot formation to occur.

Unlike the safe natural forms of vitamin K_1 and vitamin K_2 and their various isomers, a synthetic form of vitamin K, vitamin K_3 (menadione), is demonstrably toxic at high levels. The U.S. FDA has banned this form from over-the-counter sale in the United States because large doses have been shown to cause allergic reactions, hemolytic anemia, and cytotoxicity in liver cells.

Dietary Recommendations

The U.S. Institute of Medicine (IOM) updated Estimated Average Requirements (EARs) and Recommended Dietary Allowances (RDAs) for vitamin K in 1998. The IOM does not distinguish between K_1 and K_2 – both are counted as vitamin K. At that time, sufficient information was not available to establish EARs and RDAs for vitamin K. In instances such as these, the board sets Adequate Intakes (AIs), with the understanding that at some later date, AIs will be replaced by more exact information. The current AIs for adult women and men ages 19 and up are 90 and 120 µg/day, respectively. AI for pregnancy is 90 µg/day. AI for lactation is 90 µg/day. For infants up to 12 months, the AI is 2.0-2.5 µg/day; for children ages 1–18 years the AI increases with age from 30 to 75 µg/day. As for safety, the IOM sets tolerable upper intake levels (known as ULs) for vitamins and minerals when evidence is sufficient. Vitamin K has no UL, as human data for adverse effects from high doses are inadequate. Collectively, the EARs, RDAs, AIs and ULs are referred to as Dietary Reference Intakes.

The European Food Safety Authority (EFSA) refers to the collective set of information as Dietary Reference Values, with Population Reference Intake (PRI) instead of RDA, and Average Requirement instead of EAR. AI and UL are defined the same as in United States. For women and men over age 18 the AI is set at 70 µg/day. AI for pregnancy is 70 µg/day, ad for lactation 70 µg/day. For children ages 1–17 years, the AIs increase with age from 12 to 65 µg/day. These AIs are lower than the U.S. RDAs. The EFSA also reviewed the safety question and reached the same conclusion as in United States - that there was not sufficient evidence to set a UL for vitamin K.

For U.S. food and dietary supplement labeling purposes, the amount in a serving is expressed as a percentage of Daily Value (%DV). For vitamin K labeling purposes, 100% of the Daily Value was 80 µg, but as of May 27, 2016, it was revised upwards to 120 µg, to bring it into agreement with the AI. A table of the old and new adult Daily Values is provided at Reference Daily Intake. The original deadline to be in compliance was July 28, 2018, but on September 29, 2017, the FDA released a proposed rule that extended the deadline to January 1, 2020 for large companies and January 1, 2021 for small companies.

Food Sources

Vitamin K_1

Vitamin K_1 is found chiefly in leafy green vegetables such as spinach, swiss chard, lettuce and *Brassica* vegetables (such as cabbage, kale, cauliflower, broccoli, and brussels sprouts) and often the absorption is greater when accompanied by fats such as butter or oils. Some fruits, such as avocados, kiwifruit and grapes, also contain vitamin K. Some vegetable oils, notably soybean oil, contain vitamin K, but at levels that would require relatively large calorie consumption to meet the recommended amounts.

The tight binding of vitamin K_1 to thylakoid membranes in chloroplasts makes it less bioavailable. For example, cooked spinach has a 5% bioavailability of phylloquinone, however, fat added to it increases bioavailability to 13% due to the increased solubility of vitamin K in fat.

Vitamin K_2

Vitamin K_2 can be found in eggs, dairy, and meat, as well as fermented foods such as cheese and yogurt.

Deficiency

Average diets are usually not lacking in vitamin K, and primary deficiency is rare in healthy adults. Newborn infants are at an increased risk of deficiency. Other populations with an increased prevalence of vitamin K deficiency include those who suffer from liver damage or disease (e.g. alcoholics), cystic fibrosis, or inflammatory bowel diseases, or have recently had abdominal surgeries. Secondary vitamin K deficiency can occur in people with bulimia, those on stringent diets, and those taking anticoagulants. Other drugs associated with vitamin K deficiency include salicylates, barbiturates, and cefamandole, although the mechanisms are still unknown. Vitamin K deficiency has been defined as a vitamin K-responsive hypoprothrombinemia which increase prothrombin time and thus can result in coagulopathy, a bleeding disorder. Symptoms of K_1 deficiency include anemia, bruising, nosebleeds and bleeding of the gums in both sexes, and heavy menstrual bleeding in women.

Osteoporosis and coronary heart disease are strongly associated with lower levels of K_2 (menaquinone). Vitamin K_2 (as menaquinones MK-4 through MK-10) intake level is inversely related to severe aortic calcification and all-cause mortality.

Biochemistry

Function in Animals

The function of vitamin K_2 in the animal cell is to add a carboxylic acid functional group to a glutamate (Glu) amino acid residue in a protein, to form a gamma-carboxyglutamate (Gla) residue. This is a somewhat uncommon posttranslational modification of the protein, which is then known as a "Gla protein". The presence of two –COOH (carboxylic acid) groups on the same carbon in the gamma-carboxyglutamate residue allows it to chelate calcium ions. The binding of calcium ions in this way very often triggers the function or binding of Gla-protein enzymes, such as the so-called vitamin K-dependent clotting factors discussed below.

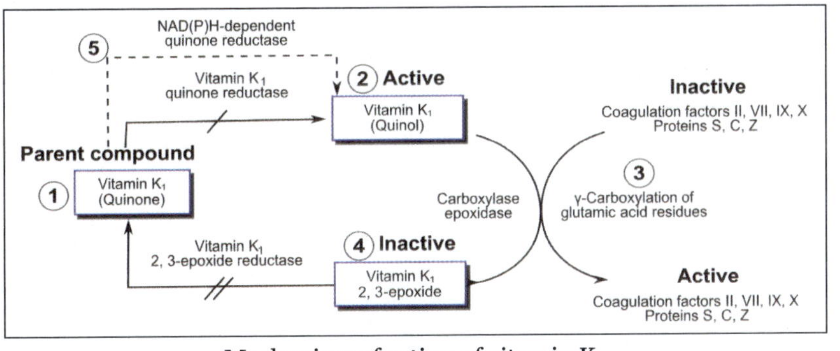

Mechanism of action of vitamin K_1.

Within the cell, vitamin K undergoes electron reduction to a reduced form called vitamin K hydroquinone, catalyzed by the enzyme vitamin K epoxide reductase (VKOR). Another enzyme then oxidizes vitamin K hydroquinone to allow carboxylation of Glu to Gla; this enzyme is called gamma-glutamyl carboxylase or the vitamin K-dependent carboxylase. The carboxylation reaction only proceeds if the carboxylase enzyme is able to oxidize vitamin K hydroquinone to vitamin K epoxide at the same time. The carboxylation and epoxidation reactions are said to be coupled. Vitamin K epoxide is then reconverted to vitamin K by VKOR. The reduction and subsequent reoxidation of vitamin K coupled with carboxylation of Glu is called the vitamin K cycle. Humans are rarely deficient in vitamin K_1 because, in part, vitamin K_1 is continuously recycled in cells.

Warfarin and other 4-hydroxycoumarins block the action of VKOR. This results in decreased concentrations of vitamin K and vitamin K hydroquinone in tissues, such that the carboxylation reaction catalyzed by the glutamyl carboxylase is inefficient. This results in the production of clotting factors with inadequate Gla. Without Gla on the amino termini of these factors, they no longer bind stably to the blood vessel endothelium and cannot activate clotting to allow formation of a clot during tissue injury. As it is impossible to predict what dose of warfarin will give the desired degree of clotting suppression, warfarin treatment must be carefully monitored to avoid overdose.

Gamma-Carboxyglutamate Proteins

The following human Gla-containing proteins ("Gla proteins") have been characterized to the level of primary structure: blood coagulation factors II (prothrombin), VII, IX, and X, anticoagulant protein C and protein S, and the factor X-targeting protein Z. The bone Gla protein osteocalcin, the calcification-inhibiting matrix Gla protein (MGP), the cell growth regulating growth arrest specific gene 6 protein (Gas6), and the four transmembrane Gla proteins (TMGPs), the function of which is at present unknown. Gas6 can function as a growth factor to activate the Axl receptor tyrosine kinase and stimulate cell proliferation or prevent apoptosis in some cells. In all cases in which their function was known, the presence of the Gla residues in these proteins turned out to be essential for functional activity.

Gla proteins are known to occur in a wide variety of vertebrates: mammals, birds, reptiles, and fish. The venom of a number of Australian snakes acts by activating the human blood-clotting system. In some cases, activation is accomplished by snake Gla-containing enzymes that bind to the endothelium of human blood vessels and catalyze the conversion of procoagulant clotting factors into activated ones, leading to unwanted and potentially deadly clotting.

Another interesting class of invertebrate Gla-containing proteins is synthesized by the fish-hunting snail *Conus geographus*. These snails produce a venom containing hundreds of neuroactive peptides, or conotoxins, which is sufficiently toxic to kill an adult human. Several of the conotoxins contain two to five Gla residues.

Methods of Assessment

Vitamin K status can be assessed by:

- The prothrombin time (PT) test measures the time required for blood to clot. A blood sample is mixed with citric acid and put in a fibrometer; delayed clot formation indicates a deficiency. This test is insensitive to mild deficiency, as the values do not change until the concentration of prothrombin in the blood has declined by at least 50%.

- Undercarboxylated prothrombin (PIVKA-II); in a study of 53 newborns, found "PT (prothrombin time) is a less sensitive marker than PIVKA II", and as indicated above, PT is unable to detect subclinical deficiencies that can be detected with PIVKA-II testing.

- Plasma phylloquinone was found to be positively correlated with phylloquinone intake in elderly British women, but not men, but an article by Schurgers *et al.* reported no correlation between responses in a food frequency questionnaire and plasma phylloquinone.

- Urinary γ-carboxyglutamic acid responds to changes in dietary vitamin K intake. Several days are required before any change can be observed. Increases of phylloquinone intakes from 100 μg to between 377 and 417 μg for five days did not induce a significant change. Response may be age-specific.

- Undercarboxylated osteocalcin (UcOc) levels have been inversely correlated with stores of vitamin K and bone strength in developing rat tibiae. Another study following 78 post-menopausal Korean women found a supplement regimen of vitamins K and D, and calcium, but not a regimen of vitamin D and calcium, was inversely correlated with reduced UcOc levels.

Function in Bacteria

Many bacteria, such as *Escherichia coli* found in the large intestine, can synthesize vitamin K_2 (menaquinone-7 or MK-7, up to MK-11), but not vitamin K_1 (phylloquinone). In these bacteria, menaquinone transfers two electrons between two different small molecules, during oxygen-independent metabolic energy production processes (anaerobic respiration). For example, a small molecule with an excess of electrons (also called an electron donor) such as lactate, formate, or NADH, with the help of an enzyme, passes two electrons to menaquinone. The menaquinone, with the help of another enzyme, then transfers these two electrons to a suitable oxidant, such fumarate or nitrate (also called an electron acceptor). Adding two electrons to fumarate or nitrate converts the molecule to succinate or nitrite plus water, respectively.

Some of these reactions generate a cellular energy source, ATP, in a manner similar to eukaryotic cell aerobic respiration, except the final electron acceptor is not molecular oxygen, but fumarate or nitrate. In aerobic respiration, the final oxidant is molecular oxygen (O_2), which accepts four electrons from an electron donor such as NADH to be converted to water. *E. coli*, as facultative anaerobes, can carry out both aerobic respiration and menaquinone-mediated anaerobic respiration.

Mineral

- Minerals are inorganic substances required by the body in small amounts for a variety of different functions.
- Minerals are involved in the formation of bones and teeth; they are essential constituents of body fluids and tissues; they are components of enzyme systems and they are involved in normal nerve function.
- The body requires different amounts of each mineral; people have different requirements, according to their age, sex, physiological state (e.g. pregnancy) and sometimes their state of health.
- The Department of Health has published Dietary Reference Values (DRVs) for minerals for different groups of healthy people.

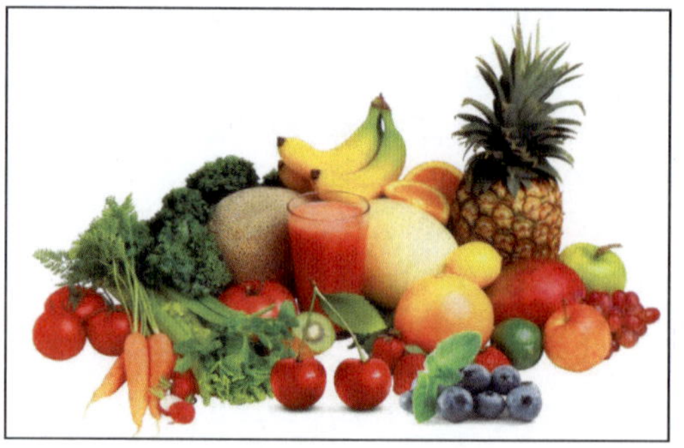

What are Minerals?

Minerals are inorganic substances required by the body in small amounts for a variety of functions. These include the formation of bones and teeth; as essential constituents of body fluids and tissues; as components of enzyme systems and for normal nerve function.

Some minerals are needed in larger amounts than others, e.g. calcium, phosphorus, magnesium, sodium, potassium and chloride. Others are required in smaller quantities and are sometimes called trace minerals, e.g. iron, zinc, iodine, fluoride, selenium and copper. Despite being required in smaller amounts, trace minerals are no less important than other minerals.

Minerals are often absorbed more efficiently by the body if supplied in foods rather than as supplements. Also, a diet that is short in one mineral may well be low in others, and so the first step in dealing with this is to review and improve the diet as a whole. Eating a varied diet will help ensure an adequate supply of most minerals for healthy people.

The National Diet and Nutrition Surveys (NDNS) have revealed that some sub-groups of the population have low intakes of some other minerals, for example potassium, magnesium, zinc in men, and for women, iron, calcium, copper and iodine. Young British adults, especially young women, have particularly poor diets which are likely to put their future health at risk unless improvements are made.

Most people do not show signs of deficiency but this does not mean their intakes or nutrient status are adequate. For example, adolescent girls, women of childbearing age and some vegans/vegetarians are more susceptible to low iron status as their dietary intake may not match their requirements, and therefore they are at risk of iron deficiency anaemia. There is also concern about the calcium intake of some adolescents, and young and older women and the implications for future bone health.

Requirements and Recommended Dietary Intakes

The body requires different amounts of each mineral because each mineral has a different set of functions. Requirements vary according to age, sex and physiological state (for example pregnancy). They may also be influenced by state of health. The Department of

Health has published recommendations in the form of Dietary Reference Values (DRVs) for minerals for different groups of healthy people. The Reference Nutrient Intake (RNI) is the amount of a nutrient that will satisfy the needs of practically all the population (i.e. 97.5%); in other words it is usually not necessary to exceed the RNI. Lower Reference Nutrient Intakes have also been established. These are levels judged to be sufficient for only 2.5% of a given population, everyone else will require more. So if, say, 10% of a population group have intakes of a nutrient below the LRNI for that nutrient, it is highly likely that the majority of these people are having insufficient for their needs.

But certain groups of people may have higher requirements for specific minerals, e.g. women with particularly heavy periods may need extra iron, and extra calcium (and vitamin D) is sometimes recommended by doctors for women at high risk of osteoporosis. In such cases, supplements may be useful but should not replace a varied and healthy diet.

The Bioavailability and Absorption of Minerals

The bioavailability of a mineral (i.e. how readily it can be absorbed and used by the body) may be influenced by a variety of factors. Bioavailability will depend upon the chemical form of the mineral, other substances present in the diet and (for nutrients such as iron) the individual person's needs as determined by how much of the nutrient is already stored in the body. This is because the body has sensitive mechanisms for preventing storage of nutrients that can be damaging in excess (as is the case with iron).

For example, the bioavailability of iron from plant sources (non-haem iron) is relatively poor compared with iron from meat (haem iron) but absorption is increased when vitamin C is consumed during the same meal because the vitamin C converts it to a more bioavailable chemical form.

Some dietary constituents reduce bioavailability. Phytate, for example, found in products made from wholegrain cereals (especially unleavened breads such as chapattis) can bind and hence reduce the absorption of calcium, iron and zinc. Iodine absorption may be hindered by nitrates. Similarly, oxalate present in spinach and rhubarb binds any calcium present, making it unavailable for absorption. Also an excess of one mineral may hinder the absorption of another by competing for the same transport systems in the gut, e.g. excess iron reduces zinc absorption. This generally only becomes a problem when zinc intakes are already marginal.

Unlike some vitamins, minerals are fairly stable in normal food processing and storage conditions.

Deficiencies and Excess Intakes

Iron deficiency anaemia is the most common nutritional deficiency in the world, often affecting women and young children, and is found in the UK population too. Iodine deficiency is also commonplace worldwide. Nutritional deficiencies of other minerals are rare in the UK (although as indicated above, dietary intakes of a number of minerals are low in sub groups of the UK population and nutritional status of individuals may therefore be affected). Policy decisions about the adequacy of current nutrient intakes in maintaining appropriate status are often hindered by the limitations of existing markers of status and also by the available information on requirements, an example being selenium.

On the other hand, excess intakes of minerals are also sometimes of concern (for example sodium, one of several risk factors associated with high blood pressure). In general, excess intakes of a range of minerals have been reported to have varying effects, ranging from no effect (e.g. no adverse effects have been reported for excess iodine intakes up to 2mg iodine/day) to severe (e.g. excess fluoride can cause skeletal fluorosis).

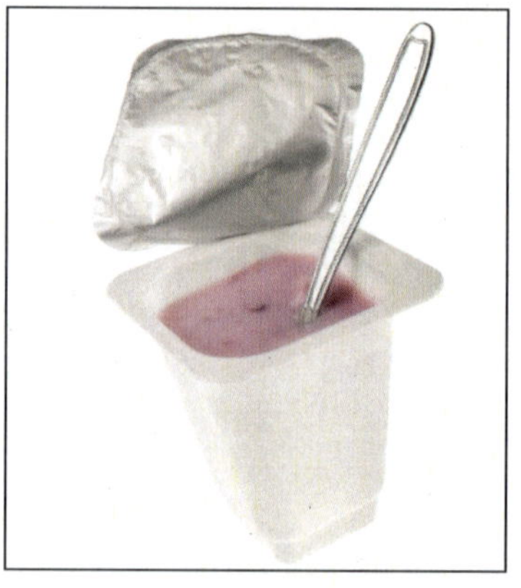

Calcium

Calcium (Ca) is the most abundant mineral in the body and is essential for a number of vital functions. The body needs adequate dietary calcium (alongside vitamin D and several other nutrients such as vitamin K) to develop and maintain healthy bones and teeth. Calcium also plays a vital role in many systems including intracellular signalling to enable the integration and regulation of metabolic processes, the transmission of information via the nervous system, the control of muscle contraction (including the heart) and blood clotting. Furthermore, it has been suggested that adequate calcium intake (for example from reduced fat dairy products) may help lower high blood pressure and may help protect against colon cancer, although more evidence is needed to fully substantiate these functions.

The skeleton contains about 99% of the body's calcium with approximately 1kg present in adult bones. The major constituents of bone are calcium and phosphate, forming hydroxyapatite, which is associated within a meshwork of collagen fibres to form a rigid structure. The body's requirement for calcium fluctuates with the rate of bone development, so as well as protecting vital organs, the skeleton acts as a 'bank' of minerals from which calcium and phosphorus may be continually withdrawn or deposited to support physiological requirement.

Calcium levels in the blood are carefully regulated and blood plasma levels are maintained within narrow limits. Calcium absorption is well controlled to match the needs of the body and so calcium balance can be maintained at a variety of different levels of calcium intake. Even at low levels of intake, there is evidence from the Gambia, for example, that calcium balance can be achieved. Calcium status is maintained by balancing calcium absorption from the gut, excretion via the kidneys and mobilisation and deposition in the bone. These sites are regulated by feedback mechanisms controlled by several hormones including parathyroid hormone and the activated form of vitamin D. Plasma levels of calcium only become abnormal if there is a breakdown of this homeostatic mechanism, and not usually as a result of differences in dietary calcium intake. The body invests this effort because small variations in plasma calcium concentrations may have serious consequences to the functioning of vital organs and to health in general. Low blood calcium is called hypocalcaemia and high blood calcium is called hypercalcaemia.

Deficiency

For some nutrients, nutritional deficiency is identified by the existence of a low blood level of the nutrient but for nutrients such as calcium, low blood levels rarely occur. Because of the need to maintain blood levels, the impact of a poor supply of calcium is usually reflected in bone density because bone acts as a reservoir in times of need. For example, insufficient calcium in bones can result from an inadequate supply of vitamin D which is essential for absorption of calcium. In children, vitamin D deficiency results in rickets and, in adults, osteomalacia, in which bones become weak owing to lack of calcium.

In terms of dietary supply, a significant proportion of young women have average calcium intakes below the Lower Reference Nutrient Intakes (8% of women aged 19-24 years and 6% of women aged 25-34 years) indicating these intakes are likely to be inadequate. An adequate calcium intake is vital for health, particularly in times of growth (in childhood, adolescence, pregnancy) to establish peak bone mass and also during lactation (breast-feeding). Supplements are sometimes recommended for those at risk of osteoporosis.

Adverse Effects

Obtaining calcium as part of a varied diet is unlikely to cause any adverse effects but taking high dose supplements sometimes causes stomach pain and diarrhoea.

Food Sources

Milk, cheese and other dairy products provide about half of the calcium in the UK diet. Bread is also an important source in the UK because most bread flour (though not wholemeal) is fortified with calcium by law. Calcium is also provided by some green leafy vegetables such as broccoli and cabbage (but not spinach), fortified soya products and fish eaten with the bones such as sardines, tinned salmon and whitebait.

Calcium Absorption

Calcium absorption is influenced by a number of promoting and inhibitory factors. Promoting factors include vitamin D, lactose, dietary protein, non-digestible oligosaccharides and an acidic environment in the small intestine. Calcium is most readily absorbed from milk and dairy products. Inhibitory factors include phytates (e.g. in wholegrain cereals, pulses), oxalate (e.g. from spinach, rhubarb, beetroot), use of antacids, unabsorbed dietary fats, excessive intakes of dietary fibre and large intakes of phosphoric acid (e.g. from carbonated drinks). Calcium is often less available from plant foods where the calcium may be bound by phytates and oxalates in foods, which makes the calcium unavailable for absorption from the intestine into the blood. However, absorption from some plant foods is good e.g. broccoli, although the amount present is usually lower than in milk.

Phosphorus

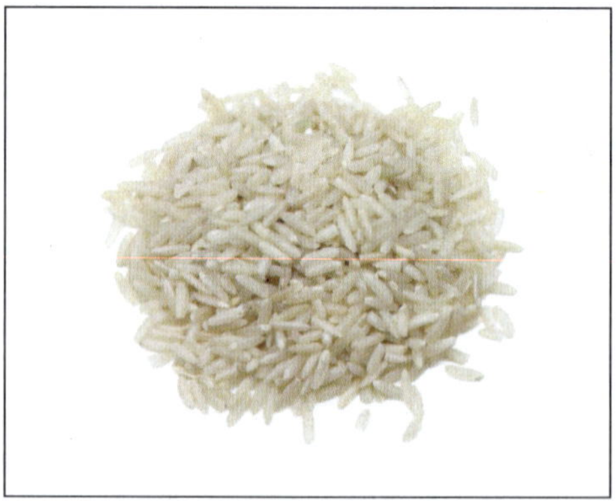

The major function of phosphorus is in the formation, with calcium, of the bone component hydroxyapatite. 80% of the phosphorous in the body is present as calcium salts in the skeleton and, therefore, is essential for healthy bone and tooth structure. In the adult, there is a dynamic equilibrium between calcium and phosphate in the continual remodelling of bones. The rest of the body's phosphorus is distributed in all cells. It is essential for the structure of cell membranes (in phospholipids) and intercellular phosphorus contributes to a number of processes associated with energy metabolism.

Deficiency

Phosphorus is unlikely to be in short supply in UK diets because it is available in many foods.

Adverse Effects

Phosphorus has very low toxicity.

Food Sources

Phosphorus is abundant in red meat, dairy products, fish, poultry, bread, rice and oats and is usually found in foods that also contain calcium.

Magnesium

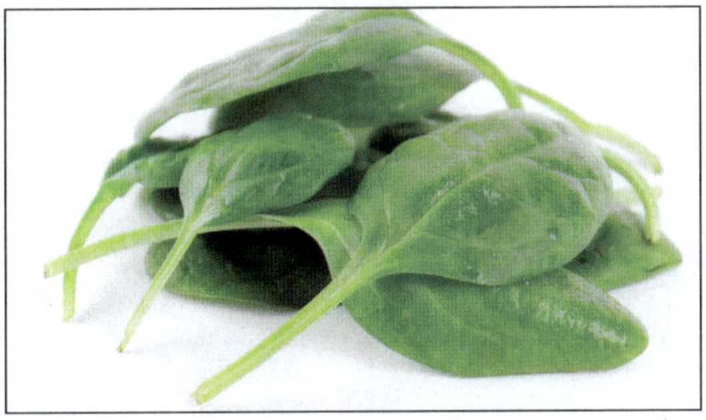

Magnesium is an essential mineral present in all human tissues, especially in bone. It has both physiological and biochemical functions and has important interrelationships with calcium, potassium and sodium. It is needed for the activation of many enzymes (for example enzymes concerned with the replication of DNA and the synthesis of RNA) and for parathyroid hormone secretion, which in involved in bone metabolism. It is also needed for muscle and nerve function.

Deficiency

Nutritional deficiency is rare and characterised by progressive muscle weakness and neuromuscular dysfunction. Mild hypomagnesaemia (low blood magnesium) is common in severely ill patients, alcoholics and those with malabsorption disorders.

In contrast, intakes of magnesium that are judged to be too low are quite common in the UK. Despite magnesium being available in a wide range of foods, one in five women aged 19-34 years and more than half of teenage girls have intakes below the LRNI (51% of 11-14 age group and 53% of 15-18 age group) and more than 20% of boys aged 11-14 years are also at risk of low intakes.

Adverse Effects

There is no evidence that large dietary intakes are harmful to humans with normal kidney function. However, regular intake of high dose supplements can result in diarrhoea and may also result in raised blood levels of magnesium with associated adverse effects.

Food Sources

Magnesium is present in both plant and animal cells and is the mineral in chlorophyll, the green pigment in plants, and so is widely available. Sources include green leafy vegetables, nuts, bread, fish, meat and dairy products.

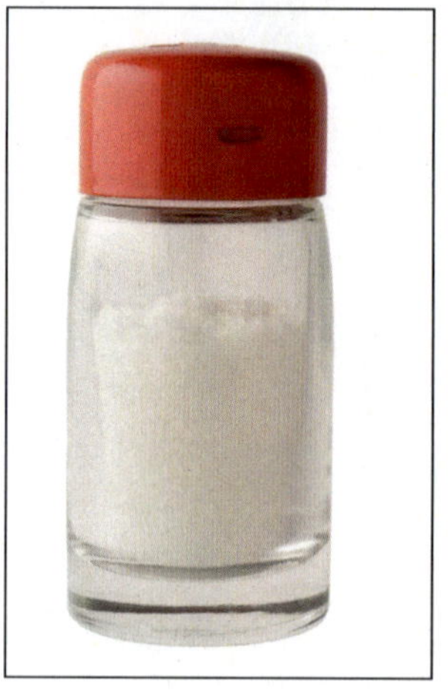

Sodium

Sodium is responsible for regulating body water content and electrolyte balance. The control of blood sodium levels depends on a balance between sodium excretion and absorption at the kidneys, which is regulated by nerves and hormones. Sodium is also required for the absorption of certain nutrients and water from the gut. Sodium is a component of common salt, known as sodium chloride (NaCl).

Deficiency

As with some other minerals, sodium levels in blood and tissues are under homeostatic control. The kidneys tightly regulate sodium concentration and can make the urine almost salt-free or excrete sodium in urine when supply is excessive. Sodium intakes in the UK are considered to be too high and so deficiency of sodium is unlikely but under some circumstances losses can occur:

- Excess sweating:, e.g. due to exercise in a hot environment, may cause some sodium depletion.
- Diarrhoea can cause fluid loss and dehydration leading to some sodium depletion.
- The kidneys normally act to protect the body's stores of sodium, but in Addison's disease failure to produce aldosterone (hormone that allows the kidneys to retain sodium and water) leads to the kidneys inability to conserve sodium.

- Renal failure: The kidneys may also lose sodium in some types of renal failure.
- Drugs: Diuretic drugs may remove large amounts of sodium in the urine.

Adverse Effects

High sodium intakes, along with obesity and high alcohol intake, are considered to be among the risk factors for high blood pressure (hypertension), which is a risk factor for cardiovascular disease and stroke. A low salt diet may be used in the treatment of hypertension.

Food Sources

Most raw foods contain very small amounts of sodium chloride (salt). But salt is often added during the processing, preparation, preservation and serving of foods. The Food Standards Agency's 2008 urinary sodium survey assessed salt intakes in the general adult population in the UK and showed that some progress had been made towards the 6g/day target for adults. The survey showed a reduction in the UK's average daily salt consumption from 9.5g to 8.6g since the National Nutrition and Diet Survey (NDNS) in 2000/01. Work continues to reduce the amount of salt present in the food supply. To date much of the emphasis has been on foods sold through supermarkets but food consumed outside the home is also beginning to be targeted by the FSA's activities.

In May 2009, the FSA published its revised salt targets for 2010 and 2012, following a review of the existing targets during 2008. The FSA emphasised the reductions that had already been achieved across the food industry: the average amount of salt in prepacked bread is down by a third; there have been reductions of the order of 44% in the salt content of branded breakfast cereal; in 2007 alone there was a 13% reduction in the salt content of standard crisps, 32% in extruded snacks and 27% in pelleted snacks (some standard crisps have been reduced by up to 55%); 30% reductions in popular brands of cooking and pasta sauces and 25% in leading brands of soups; and salt in cheeses has been reduced e.g. 50% less in a range of soft white cheeses and 32% in some standard cheese slices. In addition retailers have achieved salt reduction across a wide range of own brand products.

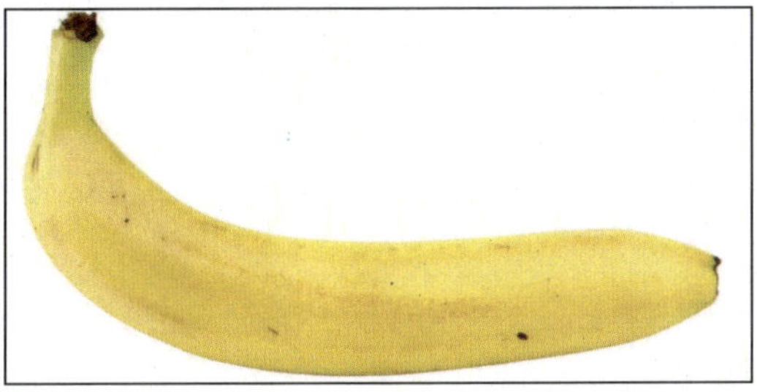

Potassium

Potassium is essential for water and electrolyte balance and the normal functioning of cells, including nerves. Increased dietary intakes of potassium have been associated with a decrease in blood pressure, as it promotes loss of sodium in the urine. It is suggested that an increase in potassium intakes may offset the impact of some of the sodium in the diet, therefore helping to protect cardiovascular health.

Deficiency

Low blood potassium levels (hypokalaemia) can result from severe diarrhoea. Symptoms include weakness, mental confusion and, if extreme, heart failure.

Low dietary potassium intakes have been observed in the UK: in the NDNS of adults about 1 in 5 women had intakes below the LRNI and in common with some other minerals, potassium intakes were lower among younger women. In the NDNS of young people, 10–15% of boys had intakes below the LRNI but among girls, about 1 in 5 11-14 year olds and about 2 in 5 15–18 year olds had intakes below the LRNI.

Adverse Effects

High supplementary doses of potassium can be harmful especially if the kidneys are not functioning properly.

Food Sources

Potassium is present in almost all foods but fruit (particularly bananas), vegetables, meat, fish, shellfish, nuts, seeds, pulses and milk are useful sources. Processed foods typically contain less than raw foods.

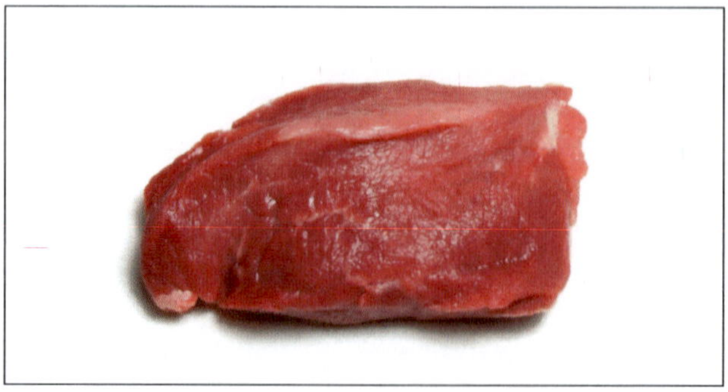

Iron

Iron is essential for the formation of haemoglobin in red blood cells; haemoglobin binds oxygen and transports it around the body. Iron is also an essential component in many enzyme reactions and has an important role in the immune system. In addition, it is required for normal energy metabolism and for the metabolism of drugs and foreign substances that need to be removed from the body.

Deficiency

A lack of dietary iron depletes iron stores in the body and this can eventually lead to iron deficiency anaemia. In particular, women of child bearing age and teenage girls need to ensure they consume adequate dietary iron because their requirements are higher than those of men of the same age. Also, loss of blood due to injury or large menstrual losses increases iron requirements in the short term. Data from the NDNS indicate that average daily iron intakes from foods are below the RNI for women in all age groups, except for older women (over the age of 54 years). A very significant proportion of younger women (2 out of 5) have intakes below the lower reference nutrient intake (LRNI) i.e. intakes that are likely to be inadequate.

Currently, there are no recommendations for increasing iron intake during pregnancy as the extra demand should be offset by pre-existing body stores, lack of menstrual blood loss and the increased intestinal absorptive capacity of the mother during the second and third trimesters of pregnancy.

More than 2 billion people worldwide suffer from iron deficiency anaemia, making it the most common nutritional deficiency condition.

Adverse Effects

As with some other minerals, under normal circumstances absorption of iron is tightly controlled as iron can have adverse effects owing to its ability to generate oxygen free radicals. However, 1 person in 200 of northern European descent is genetically predisposed to the iron loading disease haemchromatosis.

Food Sources

Dietary iron is found in two basic forms. Either as haem iron (from animal sources) or non-haem iron (from plant sources). Haem iron is the most bioavailable form of iron. However, the predominant form of iron in all diets is non-haem iron, found in cereals, vegetables, pulses, beans, nuts and fruit. Absorption of non-haem iron is affected by various factors in food. Phytate (in cereals and pulses), fibre, tannins (in tea) and calcium can all bind non-haem iron in the intestine, which reduces absorption. However, vitamin C, present in fruit and vegetables, aids the absorption of non-haem iron when eaten at the same time, as does meat.

Liver, red meat, pulses, nuts, eggs, dried fruits, poultry, fish, whole grains and dark green leafy vegetables are all sources of iron. Since the 1950s in the UK, all wheat flours (other than wholemeal) have been fortified with iron and many breakfast cereals are also fortified with iron and so contribute to iron intake, However, the nature of these foods imposes limitations on the type of iron that can be used as a fortificant and so low bio-availability may be an issue.

Trace Elements

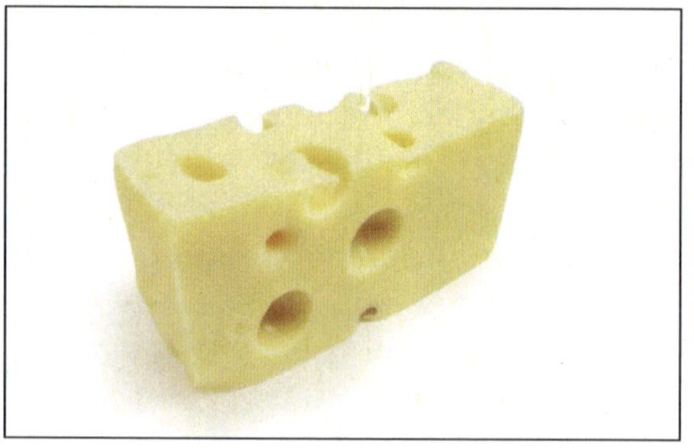

Zinc

The major function of zinc in human metabolism is as a cofactor for numerous enzymes. Zinc has a key role as a catalyst in a wide range of reactions. It is directly or indirectly involved in the major metabolic pathways concerned with protein, lipid, carbohydrate and energy metabolism and is also essential for cell division and, therefore, for growth and tissue repair and for normal reproductive development. In addition, zinc is required for the functioning of the immune system and in the structure and function of the skin, and hence plays a vital role in wound healing.

Deficiency

In some countries, delayed puberty and small stature have been linked to zinc deficiency, though it is not certain that this is due to zinc deficiency alone.

Adverse Effects

Excess zinc in the body from very high doses can interfere with copper metabolism.

Food Sources

Zinc is present in many foods and is most readily absorbed from meat, which provides about a third of zinc in the UK diet. It is also present in milk, cheese, eggs, shellfish, wholegrain cereals, nuts and pulses. For cereals and pulses, zinc's availability is limited by phytates.

Iodine

Iodine is an essential component of the thyroid hormones, thyroxine and triiodothyronine, which are vital regulators of metabolic rate and of physical and mental development.

Deficiency

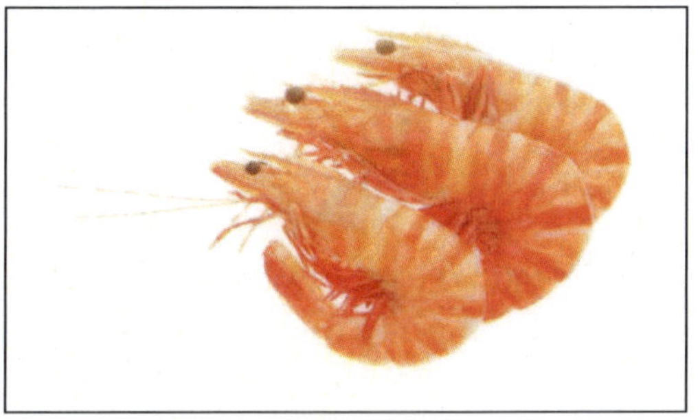

Iodine deficiency results in lethargy and swelling of the thyroid gland in the neck which forms a goitre. Iodine deficiency is relatively rare in the UK but is still prevalent in many areas of the world, where it remains a major nutritional public health issue.

Infants born of severely iodine deficient mothers may be mentally retarded (cretinism).

With regard to low dietary intakes in the UK, data from the NDNS indicate that 12% (1 in 8) young women have intakes below the LRNI. This may be associated with low intakes of milk and milk products.

Adverse Effects

Excess iodine is not absorbed so toxicity is unlikely in healthy individuals.

Food Sources

The amount of iodine in plant foods such as vegetables and cereal grains is determined by the amount of iodine in the growing plant's environment, and the amount in the soil or water can vary dramatically. The only rich sources of iodine are seafoods (sea fish, shellfish and seaweed), but milk is also a source. In some countries certain foods, e.g. salt and bread, are fortified with iodine.

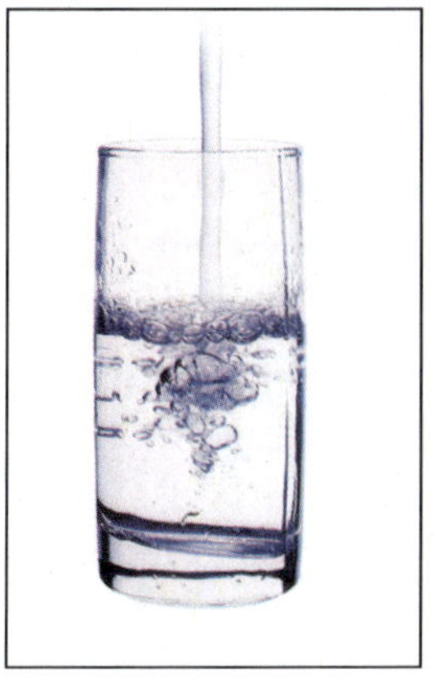

Fluoride

The main function of fluoride in the body is in the mineralisation of bones and teeth. Fluoride also protects the teeth from dental caries (tooth decay) and is now routinely added to most toothpastes.

In rare cases, very large amounts of (non-dietary) fluoride can cause fluorosis. Symptoms may be mild such as mottling and crumbling of the teeth, or more severe causing skeletal changes such as calcification of ligaments and tendons which leads to muscle, joint and bone problems.

Fluoride is found in fluoridated water, tea and fish. The diet provides only about 25% of total intake. The addition of fluoride to toothpaste is important in those areas where the water supply is low in fluoride.

Copper

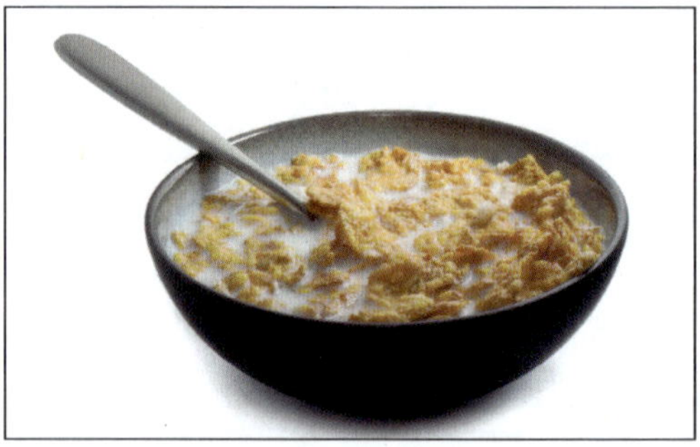

Copper is the third most abundant dietary trace metal after iron and zinc. It is a component of many enzymes and is needed to produce red and white blood cells. The body also needs copper to utilise iron efficiently and it is thought to be important for infant growth, brain development, the immune system and for strong bones.

Dietary induced copper deficiency is extremely rare due to the plentiful supply in the diet and the high efficiency of absorption. However, a rare genetic condition, known as Menke's disease, results in the inability to absorb copper and leads to severely impaired mental development, failure to keratinise hair and skeletal and vascular problems.

As with some other minerals, under normal circumstances absorption of copper is tightly controlled so overload of copper is very rare. However, Wilson's disease, another genetic condition, leads to the inability to excrete excess copper in bile and results in copper accumulation in the body, especially the liver and brain, with consequent pathological damage.

Sources of copper include shellfish, liver, kidney, nuts and wholegrain cereals (about a third of intake in the UK is from cereals).

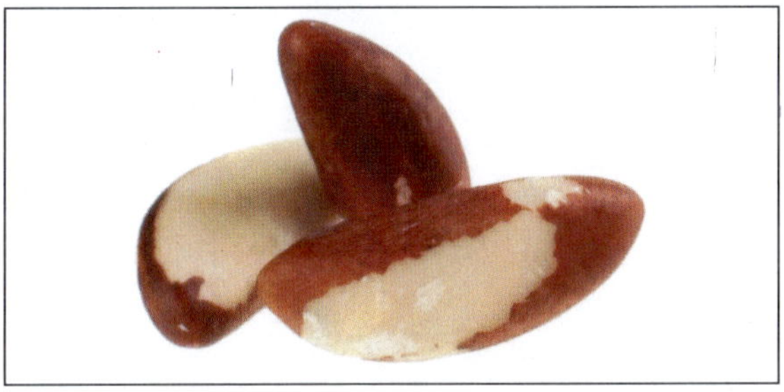

Selenium

The main function of selenium is as a component of some of the important antioxidant enzymes (e.g. glutathione peroxidase), and therefore to protect the body against oxidative damage. It is also necessary for the use of iodine in thyroid hormone production, for immune system function and for reproductive function.

The best characterised selenium deficiency condition is Keshan disease, a heart condition that affects children and women of child-bearing years in rural China where soils are deficient of selenium, leading to continuing low levels in the food chain.

Selenium intakes in the UK are below the DRVs but the implications of this are uncertain because of the lack of reliable biomarkers for selenium status and requirements.

In excess selenium is exceedingly toxic. Symptoms of selenosis (selenium excess) include brittle nails and hair, skin lesions and garlic odour on the breath.

Selenium is found in a variety of foods, especially Brazil nuts, bread, fish, meat and eggs. The selenium content of cereals is directly proportional to the selenium content in the soil. In the UK selenium intakes have fallen with the decline in import of North American selenium-rich wheat and the increased use of European cereals which are less rich in the mineral. However, some bread manufacturers still import wheat from North America.

Manganese

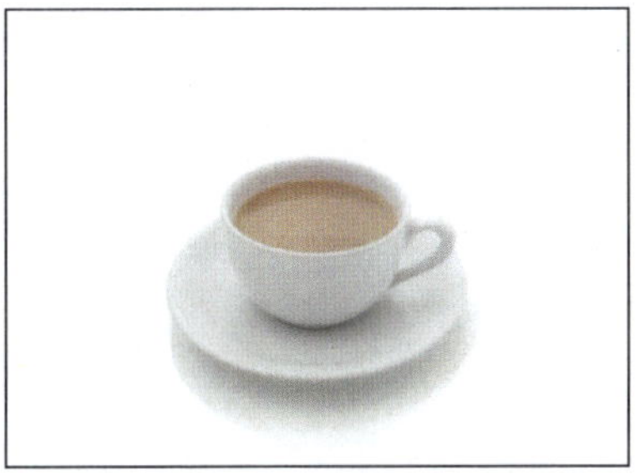

Manganese is required for bone formation and for energy metabolism. It is also a constituent of an antioxidant enzyme, which helps prevent free radical-mediated damage to cells.

Manganese deficiency is rarely seen.

Manganese toxicity is not a problem because blood levels are carefully controlled.

It is present in plant foods such as vegetables, cereals and nuts. Tea is also a rich source. In the UK, 50% of manganese intake is derived from cereals and cereal products.

Chromium

Chromium (III) is the active form of this nutrient and its main functions appear to be linked with carbohydrate and lipid metabolism. This form of chromium is thought to promote the action of insulin, the hormone which controls glucose levels in the blood. Subjects with adequate dietary chromium have improved control over blood glucose and a better blood lipid profile.

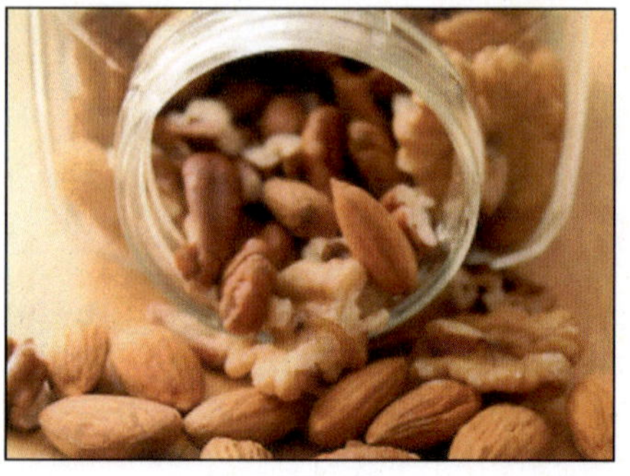

One significant characteristic of chromium deficiency is impaired glucose tolerance, which can be improved by chromium supplementation. However, chromium supplementation does not improve insulin action for people who were not initially deficient.

Chromium is not known to show toxicity.

Sources of chromium include meat, nuts, cereal grains, brewer's yeast and molasses.

Other Trace Elements

There are other minerals which are needed in tiny amounts and which appear to be essential in the diet, e.g. molybdenum, boron. Others occur in the diet, but whether they are essential is unclear, e.g. nickel, lithium, antimony, aluminium and lead.

References

- Fennema O (2008). Fennema's Food Chemistry. CRC Press Taylor & Francis. pp. 454–455. ISBN 9780849392726
- Health, symptoms-of-vitamin-b-deficiency, vitamin-b-12: healthline.com, Retrieved 09 April, 2019
- Magiorkinis E, Beloukas A, Diamantis A (April 2011). "Scurvy: past, present and future". The European Journal of Internal Medicine. 22 (2): 147–52. doi:10.1016/j.ejim.2010.10.006. PMID 21402244

- Squires VR (2011). The Role of Food, Agriculture, Forestry and Fisheries in Human Nutrition - Volume IV. EOLSS Publications. p. 121. ISBN 978184826195
- Minerals-and-trace-elements,nutrients-food-and-ingredients, nutritionscience: nutrition.org.uk, Retrieved 17 May, 2019
- Heaney RP, Holick MF (March 2011). "Why the IOM recommendations for vitamin D are deficient". Journal of Bone and Mineral Research. 26 (3): 455–7. doi:10.1002/jbmr.328. PMID 21337617

5

Role of Enzymes in Metabolism

Enzymes are large molecular biological catalysts which are responsible for increasing the rate of chemical reactions. They play a vital role in the metabolic processes by increasing the reaction rates without altering the chemical equilibrium which exists between the products and reactants. The chapter closely examines these key roles of enzymes in metabolism to provide an extensive understanding of the subject.

Enzymes are biological catalysts used to speed up biochemical reactions in living organisms. Enzymes, unlike inorganic catalysts, are big molecules or macromolecules. Most enzymes in living organisms are protein molecules, some are RNA molecules. There are myriads of chemical reactions happening in living organisms continuously, and each reaction is catalyzed by a different enzyme. The reactants of the reaction catalyzed by an enzyme are called its substrates. Since they are big molecules, enzymes have a particular 3-dimensional structure. An enzyme has a pocket called an active site, into which its substrate fits. In the active site, the substrate reaches a suitable conformation, so its bonds are broken easily and new bonds are formed, leading to the formation of the products.

Examples of Enzymes in the Body

Digestive Enzymes

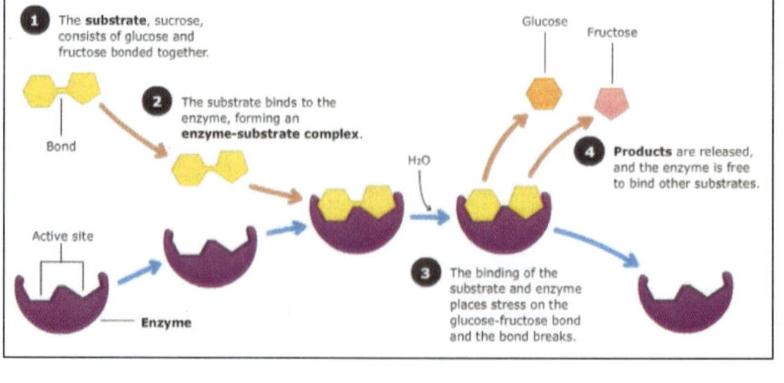

These are a group of enzymes involved in digestion of food in humans. They are:

Amylase: This enzyme helps in digestion of carbohydrates. In most cases they are break down into glucose.

The carbohydrate digestion begins in the mouth due to salivary amylase. Hence when we chew the food, it turns out to be a bit sweeter than before. This is because the salivary amylase digests starch into glucose. This glucose imparts sweetness to the taste. The remaining food is absorbed in the stomach and the intestine.

Pepsin, peptidases, Trypsin: Digests proteins into amino acids.

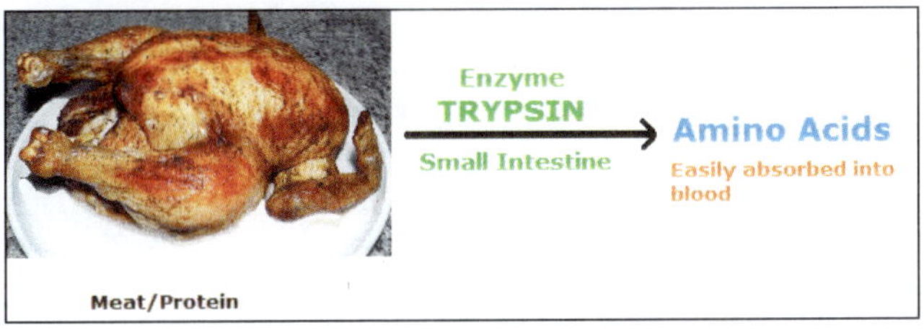

Proteins are complex molecules, and they are broken down to some extent in the stomach but to a large extent in the small intestine.

Lipase: These enzymes digest fats and oils to fatty acids and alcohols for easy absorption. This enzyme is one of the pancreatic enzymes.

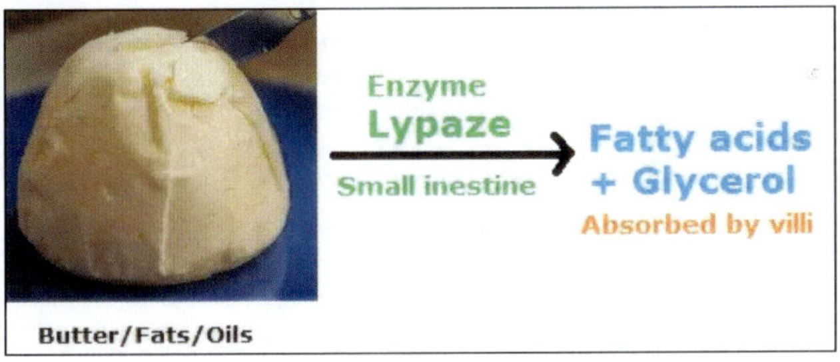

Nucleases: Breakdown nucleic acids into nucleotides.

Lysozyme is another enzyme which is present in the saliva of the mouth and this kills microbes in the mouth.

The enzymes examples mentioned are present near the gastrointestinal tract.

Receptor enzymes: These enzymes are part of the receptors system. The major examples of enzymes of this system include kinases, phosphatases. They help in many body functions related to the activation and inactivation of individual biomolecules like the glycogen, glucose, etc. These receptors act so by either phosphorylation or dephosphorylation. Those enzymes which help in phosphorylation are called kinases and those involved in dephosphorylations are called as phosphatases. These receptors are classified under kinase-linked receptors. So few enzymes are also receptors.

Metabolic Enzymes

As the name indicates, these are the enzymes which aid in metabolism and also detoxification of substances in the body. They are like:

1. Oxidases: These oxidase substances to alcohols or ketones etc.
2. Hydrolases: These breakdown materials by the addition of water.
3. Reductases: These add hydrogen to substrates in the reaction.
4. Lyases: The enzymes which are involved in breaking of molecules without hydrolysis or oxidation.
5. Ligases: Enzymes which brings in a bonding of two or more molecules.
6. Isomerases: These enzymes convert the same molecule from one form to another and vice versa.
7. Glucuronidase: This is the key enzyme which adds glucuronic acid to the non-water soluble substances and converts them to water-soluble forms to be excreted in urine.
8. Transaminases: These are the enzymes involved in the addition or removal of amino acids.
9. Glycogen synthase: This is the enzyme which synthesizes glycogen from glucose to store in the liver.
10. Aminoacyl tRNA synthetase: This enzyme bind amino-acid to tRNA.
11. Lactate dehydrogenase: Enzymes which converts lactate to pyruvic acid.

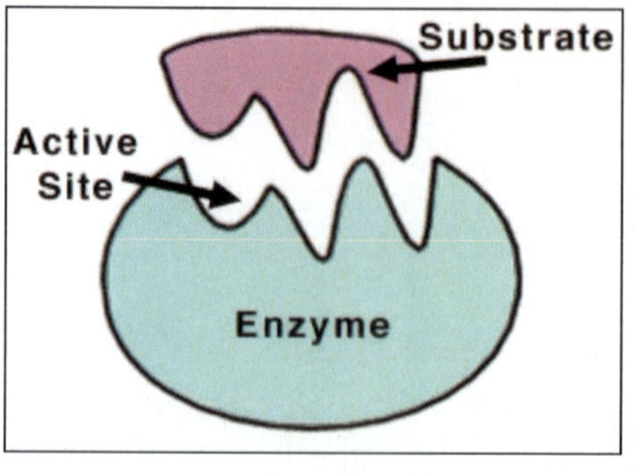

Liver enzymes: Liver is an organ of metabolism in the body. It detoxifies almost any substance and helps in expulsion from body through urine. There are many enzymes in liver and few of the important include:

1. SGOT is also called as aspartate aminotransferase (AST).

2. SGPT also called as Alanine transaminase (ALT). Both the enzymes catalyze amino-acids.

Both SGOT and SGPT catalyze reactions involving amino-acids.

Besides them there is a big family of metabolic enzymes named as cytochrome-P 450's. They are mainly involved in metabolism of xenobiotics. These enzymes have genetic variations among few American population (hispanics) which leads to variation in drug effects in the body. i.e., the same drug can be toxic or ineffective to one person while it is perfectly good for others.

Enzymes of nervous system: These are the ones which help in metabolism of neurotransmitters.

Example:

Acetyl cholinesterase: Breaks down acetyl choline.

Monoamine oxidase: Breaks down catecholamines like dopamine, adrenalin and nor-adrenalin.

Special enzymes in body:

1. Urokinase: Helps to breakdown clots in the body.
2. Hyaluronidase: An enzyme secreted by sperm when released into female reproductive tract. This enzyme helps pierce through ova wall and merge with ova.
3. DNA topoisomerase-II: The enzyme which catalyses cutting (nicking) and sealing function on DNA.
4. DNA dependent RNA polymerase: An enzyme which helps in formation of mRNA.
5. Endonucleases: These are the enzymes which helps in cutting DNA strands. Restriction endonucleases are the type which cut DNA strands at one specific site. These are highly used in genetic engineering.
6. Cyclo-oxygenase Enzyme: These enzymes are of two types as COX-1 and COX-II. They regulate synthesis of prostaglanding which are involved in inflammation and gastric mucus production.

Roles Enzymes Play in Metabolism

Formation of macromolecules: Enzymes help in the creation of macro-molecules as required by the body. These macromolecules are used for regular physiology or storage.

Examples include:

a) Conversion of glucose to glycogen by the enzyme glycogen synthase. This glycogen is stored in the liver for future use.

b) Conversion of amino acids to peptides by peptide bond formation due to the enzyme peptide synthetases.

c) Formation of DNA and RNA by polymerases.

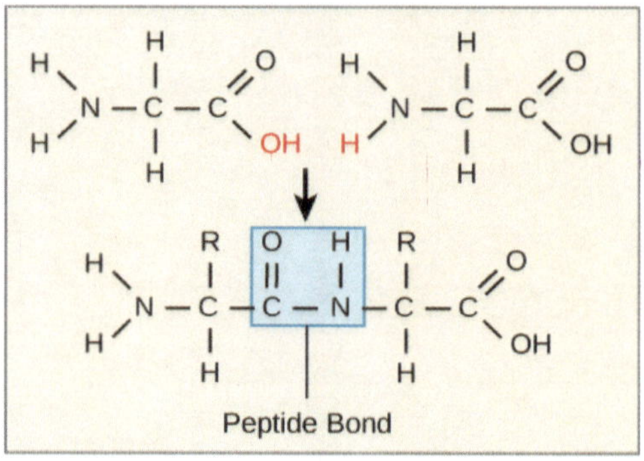

Change in the form of molecules: Molecules with the same number of elements in the structure can have different shapes and properties. In one form they can be active while in another form inactive.

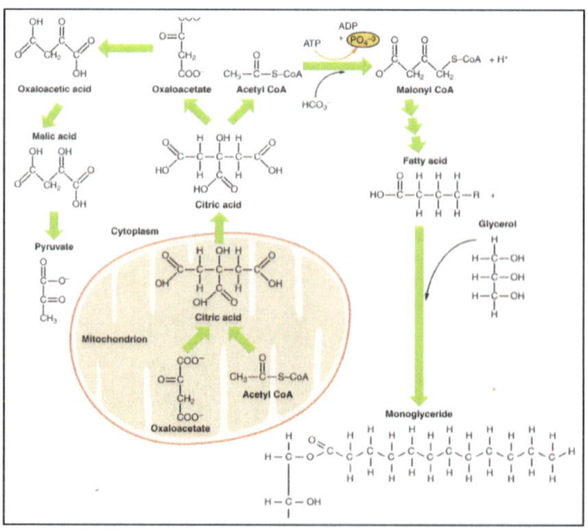

In the image above, you can notice Oxaloacetic acid converts Malic acid. Both are similar in terms of chemistry. Thus, these molecules are inter-converted based on the requirement by the enzymes like isomerases.

Breakdown of large to small molecules: Enzymes are also involved in the breakdown of large molecules to small molecules to meet the needs of the body and also for excretion from the body.

Examples:

a) Starch is broken down to release glucose in the gut in the presence of digestive enzyme amylase.

b) Glycogen is broken down into glucose by the enzyme glycogen phosphorylase.

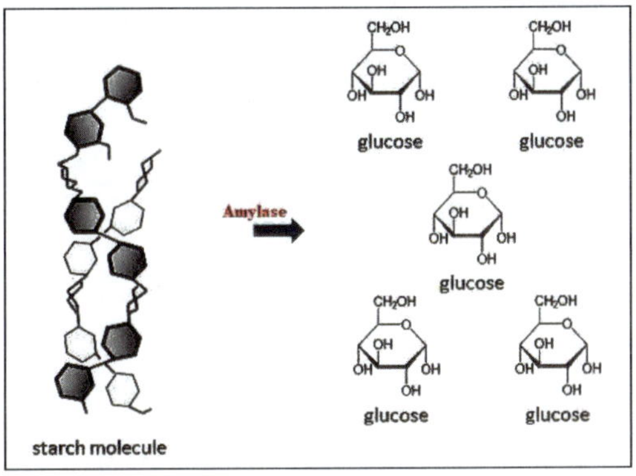

Enhancing the solubility or Convert lipophilic molecules to hydrophilic ones: When a substance is lipophilic, it tends to be distributed in the tissues and cells. When it is hydrophilic, it tries to stay in the water compartment of the body, i.e., blood and other fluids. When a substance is hydrophilic, it can be easily expelled in urine.

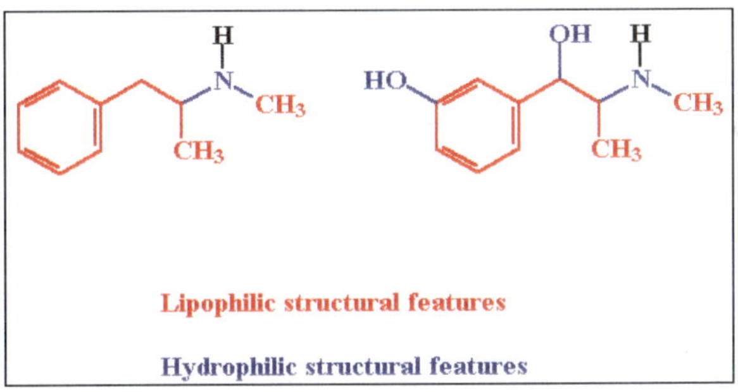

Hence, lipophilic substances are converted to hydrophilic ones by enzyme action. One common example of such reaction is glucuronidation.

Minimizing the toxicity of substances: When a substance is toxic to the body due to its chemical nature, it is metabolized by enzymes to no toxic one.

Catalytic Activity of Enzymes

Like all other catalysts, enzymes are characterized by two fundamental properties. First, they increase the rate of chemical reactions without themselves being consumed or permanently altered by the reaction. Second, they increase reaction rates without altering the chemical equilibrium between reactants and products.

These principles of enzymatic catalysis are illustrated in the following example, in which a molecule acted upon by an enzyme is converted to a product (P) as the result of the reaction. In the absence of the enzyme, the reaction can be written as follows:

$$S \rightleftharpoons P$$

The chemical equilibrium between S and P is determined by the laws of thermodynamics and is represented by the ratio of the forward and reverse reaction rates (S→P and P→S, respectively). In the presence of the appropriate enzyme, the conversion of S to P is accelerated, but the equilibrium between S and P is unaltered. Therefore, the enzyme must accelerate both the forward and reverse reactions equally. The reaction can be written as follows:

$$S \overset{E}{\rightleftharpoons} P$$

Note that the enzyme (E) is not altered by the reaction, so the chemical equilibrium remains unchanged, determined solely by the thermodynamic properties of S and P.

The effect of the enzyme on such a reaction is best illustrated by the energy changes that must occur during the conversion of S to P. The equilibrium of the reaction is determined by the final energy states of S and P, which are unaffected by enzymatic catalysis. In order for the reaction to proceed, however, the substrate must first be converted to a higher energy state, called the transition state. The energy required to reach the transition state (the activation energy) constitutes a barrier to the progress of the reaction, limiting the rate of the reaction. Enzymes (and other catalysts) act by reducing the activation energy, thereby increasing the rate of reaction. The increased rate is the same in both the forward and reverse directions, since both must pass through the same transition state.

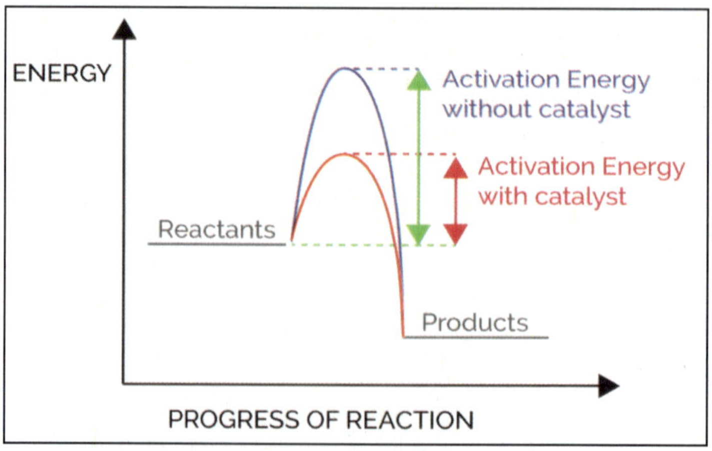

Energy diagrams for catalyzed and uncatalyzed reactions.

The reaction illustrated is the simple conversion of a substrate S to a product P. Because the final energy state of P is lower than that of S, the reaction proceeds from left to right. For the reaction to occur, however, S must first pass through a higher energy transition state. The energy required to reach this transition state (the activation energy) represents a barrier to the progress of the reaction and thereby determines the rate at which the reaction proceeds. In the presence of a catalyst (e.g., an enzyme), the activation energy is lowered and the reaction proceeds at an accelerated rate.

The catalytic activity of enzymes involves the binding of their substrates to form an enzyme-substrate complex (ES). The substrate binds to a specific region of the enzyme, called the active site. While bound to the active site, the substrate is converted into the product of the reaction, which is then released from the enzyme. The enzyme-catalyzed reaction can thus be written as follows:

$$S + E \rightleftharpoons ES \rightleftharpoons E + P$$

Note that E appears unaltered on both sides of the equation, so the equilibrium is unaffected. However, the enzyme provides a surface upon which the reactions converting S to P can occur more readily. This is a result of interactions between the enzyme and substrate that lower the energy of activation and favor formation of the transition state.

Mechanisms of Enzymatic Catalysis

The binding of a substrate to the active site of an enzyme is a very specific interaction. Active sites are clefts or grooves on the surface of an enzyme, usually composed of amino acids from different parts of the polypeptide chain that are brought together in the tertiary structure of the folded protein. Substrates initially bind to the active site by noncovalent interactions, including hydrogen bonds, ionic bonds, and hydrophobic interactions. Once a substrate is bound to the active site of an enzyme, multiple mechanisms can accelerate its conversion to the product of the reaction.

Most biochemical reactions involve interactions between two or more different substrates. For example, the formation of a peptide bond involves the joining of two amino acids. For such reactions, the binding of two or more substrates to the active site in the proper position and orientation accelerates the reaction . The enzyme provides a template upon which the reactants are brought together and properly oriented to favor the formation of the transition state in which they interact.

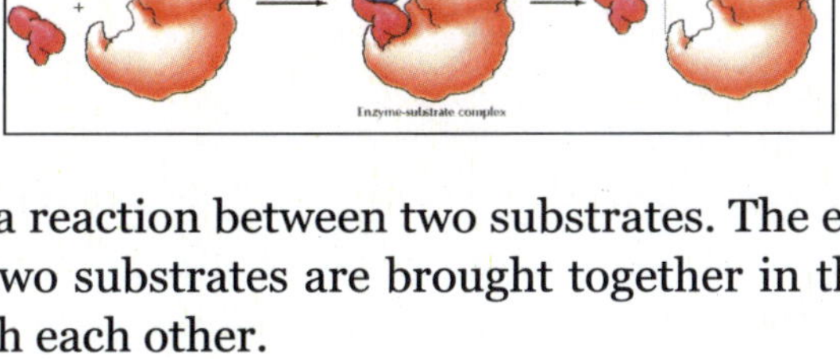

Enzymatic catalysis of a reaction between two substrates. The enzyme provides a template upon which the two substrates are brought together in the proper position and orientation to react with each other.

Enzymes accelerate reactions also by altering the conformation of their substrates to approach that of the transition state. The simplest model of enzyme-substrate interaction is the lock-and-key model, in which the substrate fits precisely into the active site. In many cases, however, the configurations of both the enzyme and substrate are modified by substrate binding—a process called induced fit. In such cases the conformation of the substrate is altered so that it more closely resembles that of the transition state. The stress produced by such distortion of the substrate can further facilitate its conversion to the transition state by weakening critical bonds. Moreover, the transition state is stabilized by its tight binding to the enzyme, thereby lowering the required energy of activation.

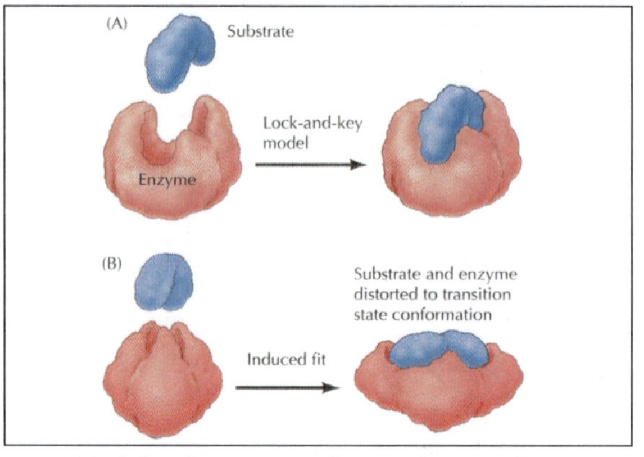

Models of enzyme-substrate interaction.

(A) In the lock-and-key model, the substrate fits precisely into the active site of the enzyme. (B) In the induced-fit model, substrate binding distorts the conformations of both substrate and enzyme. This distortion brings the substrate closer to the conformation of the transition state, thereby accelerating the reaction.

In addition to bringing multiple substrates together and distorting the conformation of substrates to approach the transition state, many enzymes participate directly in the catalytic process. In such cases, specific amino acid side chains in the active site may react with the substrate and form bonds with reaction intermediates. The acidic and basic amino acids are often involved in these catalytic mechanisms, as illustrated in the following discussion of chymotrypsin as an example of enzymatic catalysis.

Chymotrypsin is a member of a family of enzymes (serine proteases) that digest proteins by catalyzing the hydrolysis of peptide bonds. The reaction can be written as follows:

$$Protein + H_2O \rightarrow Peptide_1 + Peptide_2$$

The different members of the serine protease family (including chymotrypsin, trypsin, elastase, and thrombin) have distinct substrate specificities; they preferentially cleave peptide bonds adjacent to different amino acids. For example, whereas chymotrypsin digests bonds adjacent to hydrophobic amino acids, such as tryptophan and phenylalanine, trypsin digests bonds next to basic amino acids, such as lysine and arginine. All the serine proteases, however, are similar in structure and use the same mechanism of catalysis. The active sites of these enzymes contain three critical amino acids—serine, histidine, and aspartate—that drive hydrolysis of the peptide bond. Indeed, these enzymes are called serine proteases because of the central role of the serine residue.

Substrates bind to the serine proteases by insertion of the amino acid adjacent to the cleavage site into a pocket at the active site of the enzyme. The nature of this pocket determines the substrate specificity of the different members of the serine protease family. For example, the binding pocket of chymotrypsin contains hydrophobic amino acids that interact with the hydrophobic side chains of its preferred substrates. In contrast, the binding pocket of trypsin contains a negatively charged acidic amino acid (aspartate), which is able to form an ionic bond with the lysine or arginine residues of its substrates.

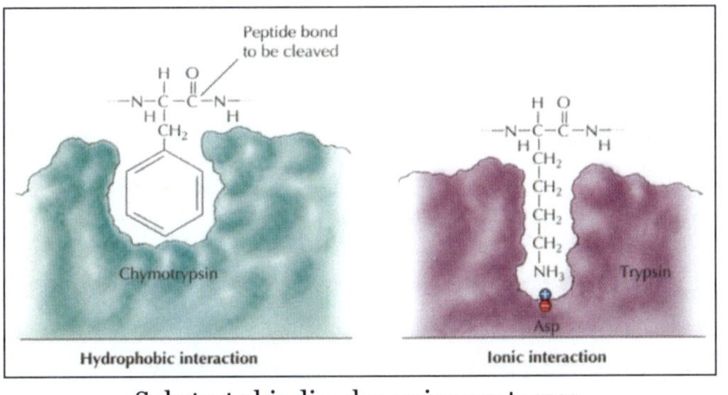

Substrate binding by serine proteases.

The amino acid adjacent to the peptide bond to be cleaved is inserted into a pocket at the active site of the enzyme. In chymotrypsin, the pocket binds hydrophobic amino acids; the binding pocket of trypsin contains a negatively charged aspartate residue that binds basic amino acids via an ionic interaction.

Substrate binding positions the peptide bond to be cleaved adjacent to the active site serine. The proton of this serine is then transferred to the active site histidine. The conformation of the active site favors this proton transfer because the histidine interacts with the negatively charged aspartate residue. The serine reacts with the substrate, forming a tetrahedral transition state. The peptide bond is then cleaved, and the C-terminal portion of the substrate is released from the enzyme. However, the N-terminal peptide remains bound to serine. This situation is resolved when a water molecule (the second substrate) enters the active site and reverses the preceding reactions. The proton of the water molecule is transferred to histidine, and its hydroxyl group is transferred to the peptide, forming a second tetrahedral transition state. The proton is then transferred from histidine back to serine, and the peptide is released from the enzyme, completing the reaction.

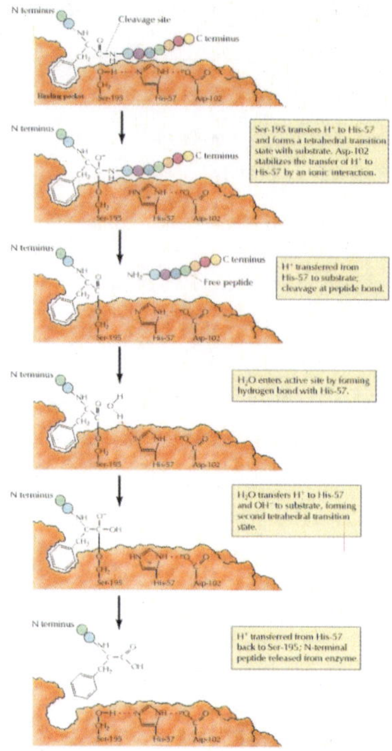

Catalytic mechanism of chymotrypsin. Three amino acids at the active site (Ser-195, His-57, and Asp-102) play critical roles in catalysis.

This example illustrates several features of enzymatic catalysis; the specificity of enzyme-substrate interactions, the positioning of different substrate molecules in the active site, and the involvement of active-site residues in the formation and stabilization of the transition state. Although the thousands of enzymes in cells catalyze many different types of chemical reactions, the same basic principles apply to their operation.

Coenzymes

In addition to binding their substrates, the active sites of many enzymes bind other small molecules that participate in catalysis. Prosthetic groups are small molecules bound to proteins in which they play critical functional roles. For example, the oxygen carried by myoglobin and hemoglobin is bound to heme, a prosthetic group of these proteins. In many cases metal ions (such as zinc or iron) are bound to enzymes and play central roles in the catalytic process. In addition, various low-molecular-weight organic molecules participate in specific types of enzymatic reactions. These molecules are called coenzymes because they work together with enzymes to enhance reaction rates. In contrast to substrates, coenzymes are not irreversibly altered by the reactions in which they are involved. Rather, they are recycled and can participate in multiple enzymatic reactions.

Coenzymes serve as carriers of several types of chemical groups. A prominent example of a coenzyme is nicotinamide adenine dinucleotide (NAD^+), which functions as a carrier of electrons in oxidation-reduction reactions. NAD^+ can accept a hydrogen ion (H^+) and two electrons (e^-) from one substrate, forming NADH. NADH can then donate these electrons to a second substrate, re-forming NAD^+. Thus, NAD^+ transfers electrons from the first substrate (which becomes oxidized) to the second (which becomes reduced).

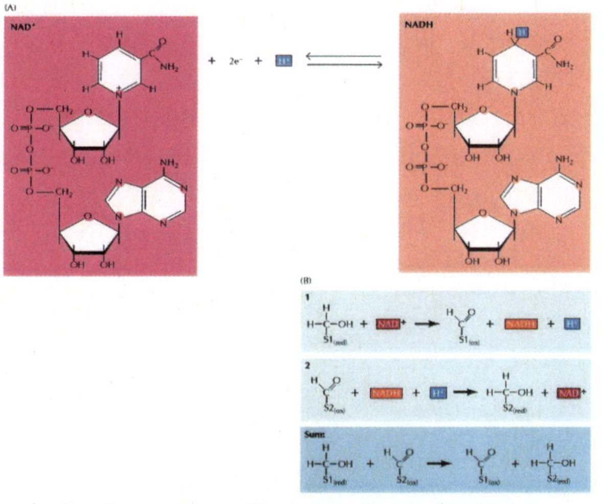

Role of NAD^+ in Oxidation-reduction Reactions.

(A) Nicotinamide adenine dinucleotide (NAD^+) acts as a carrier of electrons in oxidation-reduction reactions by accepting electrons (e^-) to form NADH. (B) For example, NAD^+ can accept electrons from one substrate (S1), yielding oxidized S1 plus NADH. The NADH formed in this reaction can then transfer its electrons to a second substrate (S2), yielding reduced S2 and regenerating NAD^+. The net effect is the transfer of electrons (carried by NADH) from S1 (which becomes oxidized) to S2 (which becomes reduced).

Several other coenzymes also act as electron carriers, and still others are involved in the transfer of a variety of additional chemical groups (e.g., carboxyl groups and acyl groups). The same coenzymes function together with a variety of different enzymes to catalyze the transfer of specific chemical groups between a wide range of substrates. Many coenzymes are closely related to vitamins, which contribute part or all of the structure of the coenzyme. Vitamins are not required by bacteria such as E. coli but are necessary components of the diets of human and other higher animals, which have lost the ability to synthesize these compounds.

Regulation of Enzyme Activity

An important feature of most enzymes is that their activities are not constant but instead can be modulated. That is, the activities of enzymes can be regulated so that they function appropriately to meet the varied physiological needs that may arise during the life of the cell.

One common type of enzyme regulation is feedback inhibition, in which the product of a metabolic pathway inhibits the activity of an enzyme involved in its synthesis. For example, the amino acid isoleucine is synthesized by a series of reactions starting from the amino acid threonine. The first step in the pathway is catalyzed by the enzyme threonine deaminase, which is inhibited by isoleucine, the end product of the pathway. Thus, an adequate amount of isoleucine in the cell inhibits threonine deaminase, blocking further synthesis of isoleucine. If the concentration of isoleucine decreases, feedback inhibition is relieved, threonine deaminase is no longer inhibited, and additional isoleucine is synthesized. By so regulating the activity of threonine deaminase, the cell synthesizes the necessary amount of isoleucine but avoids wasting energy on the synthesis of more isoleucine than is needed.

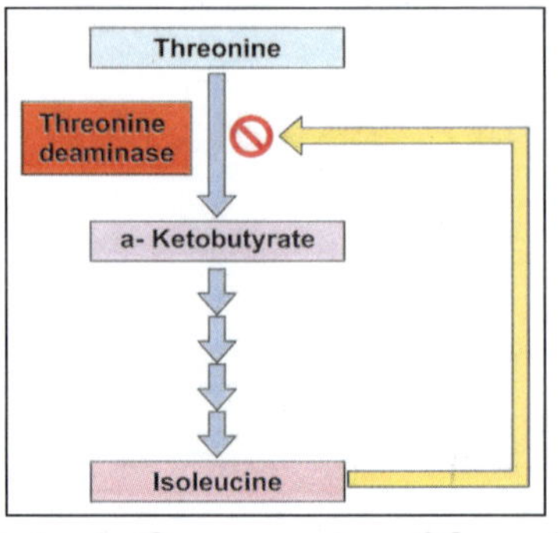

Feedback inhibition: The first step in the conversion of threonine to iso-leucine is catalyzed by the enzyme threonine deaminase. The activity of this enzyme is inhibited by isoleucine, the end product of the pathway.

Feedback inhibition is one example of allosteric regulation, in which enzyme activity is controlled by the binding of small molecules to regulatory sites on the enzyme. The term "allosteric regulation" derives from the fact that the regulatory molecules bind not to the catalytic site, but to a distinct site on the protein (allo= "other" and steric= "site"). Binding of the regulatory molecule changes the conformation of the protein, which in turn alters the shape of the active site and the catalytic activity of the enzyme. In the case of threonine deaminase, binding of the regulatory molecule (isoleucine) inhibits enzymatic activity. In other cases regulatory molecules serve as activators, stimulating rather than inhibiting their target enzymes.

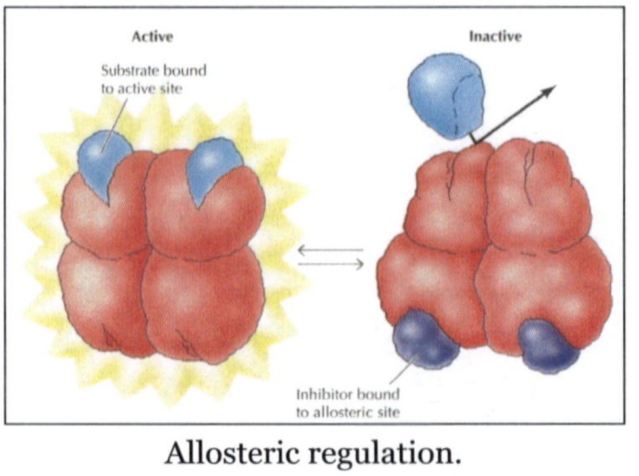

Allosteric regulation.

In this example, enzyme activity is inhibited by the binding of a regulatory molecule to an allosteric site. In the absence of inhibitor, the substrate binds to the active site of the enzyme and the reaction proceeds. The binding of inhibitor to the allosteric site induces a conformational change in the enzyme and prevents substrate binding. Most allosteric enzymes consist of multiple subunits.

The activities of enzymes can also be regulated by their interactions with other proteins and by covalent modifications, such as the addition of phosphate groups to serine, threonine, or tyrosine residues. Phosphorylation is a particularly common mechanism for regulating enzyme activity; the addition of phosphate groups either stimulates or inhibits the activities of many different enzymes. For example, muscle cells respond to epinephrine (adrenaline) by breaking down glycogen into glucose, thereby providing a source of energy for increased muscular activity. The breakdown of glycogen is catalyzed by the enzyme glycogen phosphorylase, which is activated by phosphorylation in response to the binding of epinephrine to a receptor on the surface of the muscle cell. Protein phosphorylation plays a central role in controlling not only metabolic reactions but also many other cellular functions, including cell growth and differentiation.

Factors Affecting Enzyme Activity

Biochemical reactions are necessary for growth, repairing damaged tissues, and obtaining energy and they take place in all living organisms' bodies. These reactions are called 'metabolism' and they happen all the time in living organisms. If they stop working, this leads to the death of the organism.

All the reactions that occur in living organisms require high activation energy to take place. To reduce the cell's consumption of energy, there is a catalyst to ensure that the chemical reactions occur rapidly and reduce the activation of energy. This catalyst is the enzymes.

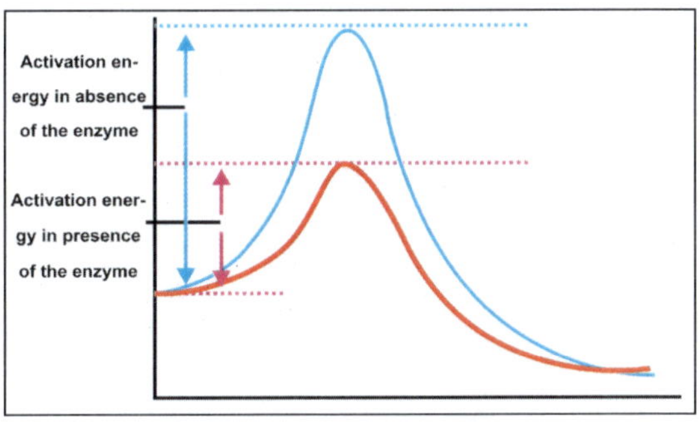

Enzyme activation energy.

Enzymes are biological catalysts made up of large protein molecules. They speed up the chemical reactions inside the cell. The enzyme is made up of a combination of amino acids which for a chain of polypeptides between each other.

Enzymes are similar to other chemical catalysts. They participate in the reaction without getting affected. In other words, they speed up the chemical reactions inside the cells without getting consumed. Enzymes are affected by the hydrogen ion concentration (pH) and the temperature. Enzymes are highly specific compared to other catalysts, and each enzyme is specialized for one reactant substance. This reactant substance is called substrate, and it is specialized for one type of reaction or a few reactions. Enzymes lower the activation energy required to get the reaction started. Collectively, these are the most important properties of the enzyme.

There are several factors that affect the speed of an enzyme's action, such as the concentration of the enzyme, the concentration of the substrate, temperature, hydrogen ion concentration (pH), and the presence of inhibitors.

Factor 1: Concentration of Enzyme

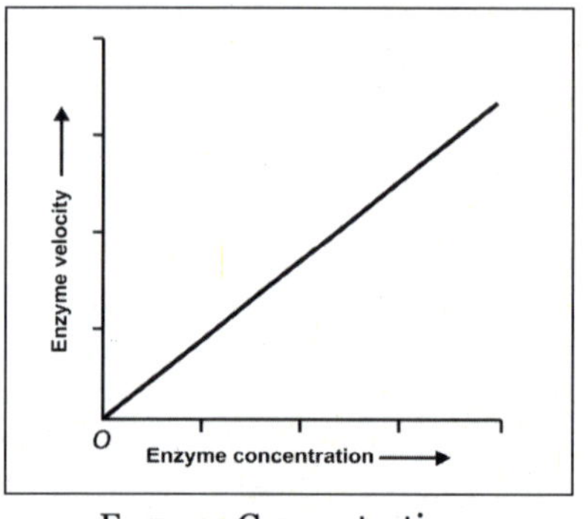

Enzyme Concentration.

As the concentration of the enzyme is increased, the velocity of the reaction proportionately increases. This property is used for determining the activities of serum enzymes during the diagnosis of diseases.

Factor 2: Concentration of Substrate

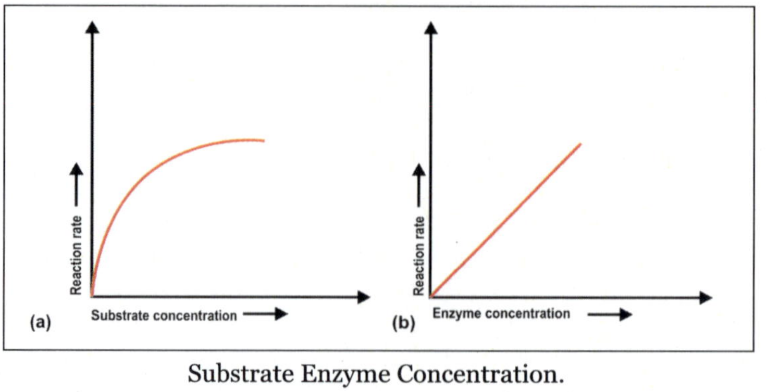

Substrate Enzyme Concentration.

In the presence of a given amount of enzyme, the rate of enzymatic reaction increases as the substrate concentration increases until a limiting rate is reached, after which further increase in the substrate concentration produces no significant change in the reaction rate. At this point, so much substrate is present that essentially all of the enzyme active sites have substrate bound to them.

In other words, the enzyme molecules are saturated with substrate. The excess substrate molecules cannot react until the substrate already bound to the enzymes has reacted and been released (or been released without reacting).

Factor 3: Effect of Temperature

The protein nature of the enzymes makes them extremely sensitive to thermal changes. Enzyme activity occurs within a narrow range of temperatures compared to ordinary chemical reactions. each enzyme has a certain temperature at which it is more active. This point is called the optimal temperature, which ranges between 37 to 40 °C.

The enzyme activity gradually lowers as the temperature rises more than the optimal temperature until it reaches a certain temperature at which the enzyme activity stops completely due to the change of its natural composition.

On the other hand, if the temperature lowers below the optimal temperature, the enzyme activity lowers until the enzyme reaches a minimum temperature at which the enzyme activity is the least. The enzyme activity stops completely at 0 °C, but if the temperature rises again, then the enzyme gets reactivated once more.

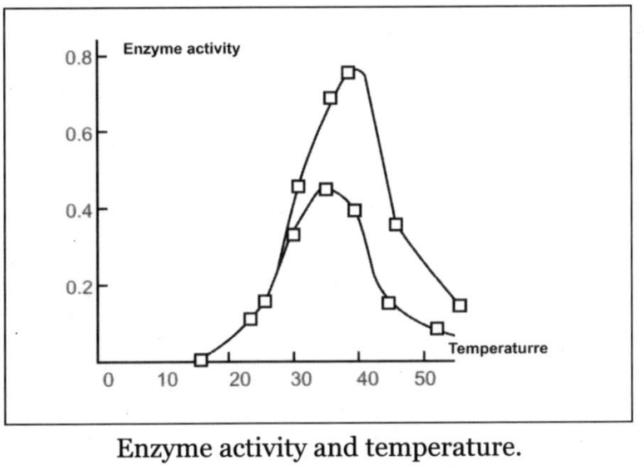

Enzyme activity and temperature.

Factor 4: Effect of pH

The potential of hydrogen (pH) is the best measurement for determining the concentration of hydrogen ion (H^+) in a solution. It also determines whether the liquid is acidic, basic or neutral. Generally, all liquids with a pH below 7 are called acids, whereas liquids with a pH above 7 are called bases or alkalines. Liquids with pH 7 are neutral and equal the acidity of pure water at 25 °C. You can determine pH of any solution using the pH indicators.

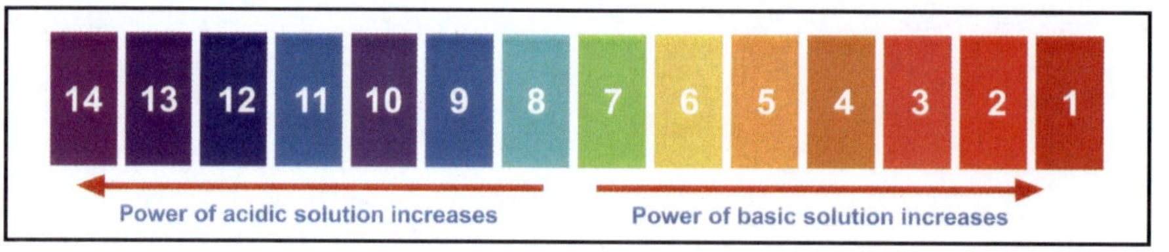

pH Indicators.

Enzymes are protein substances that contain acidic carboxylic groups ($COOH^-$) and basic amino groups (NH_2). So, the enzymes are affected by changing the pH value.

Each enzyme has a pH value that it works at with maximum efficiency called the optimal pH. If the pH is lower or higher than the optimal pH, the enzyme activity decreases until it stops working. For example, pepsin works at a low pH, i.e, it is highly acidic, while trypsin works at a high pH, i.e, it is basic. Most enzymes work at neutral pH 7.4.

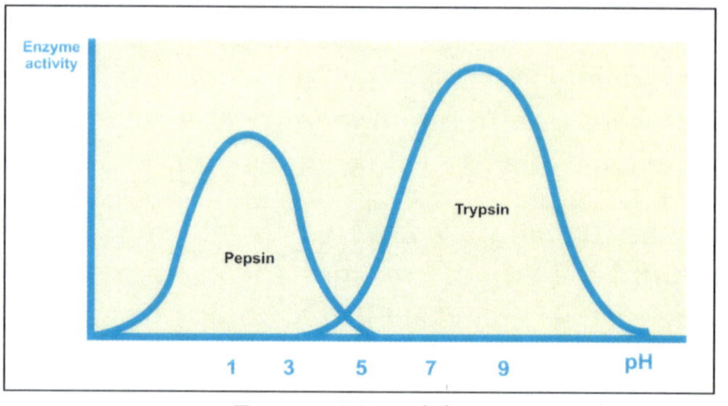

Enzyme PH activity.

Factor 5: Effect of Activators

Some of the enzymes require certain inorganic metallic cations, like Mg^{2+}, Mn^{2+}, Zn^{2+}, Ca^{2+}, Co^{2+}, Cu^{2+}, Na^+, K^+ etc., for their optimum activity. Rarely, anions are also needed for enzyme activity, e.g. a chloride ion (Cl^-) for amylase.

References

- Enzymes-classification: byjus.com, Retrieved 11 March, 2019
- Examples-of-enzymes: studyread.com, Retrieved 27 July, 2019
- What-role-do-enzymes-play-in-metabolism: studyread.com, Retrieved 09 April, 2019
- Factors-affecting-enzyme-activity: alevelbiology.co.uk, Retrieved 23 January, 2019

Permissions

All chapters in this book are published with permission under the Creative Commons Attribution Share Alike License or equivalent. Every chapter published in this book has been scrutinized by our experts. Their significance has been extensively debated. The topics covered herein carry significant information for a comprehensive understanding. They may even be implemented as practical applications or may be referred to as a beginning point for further studies.

We would like to thank the editorial team for lending their expertise to make the book truly unique. They have played a crucial role in the development of this book. Without their invaluable contributions this book wouldn't have been possible. They have made vital efforts to compile up to date information on the varied aspects of this subject to make this book a valuable addition to the collection of many professionals and students.

This book was conceptualized with the vision of imparting up-to-date and integrated information in this field. To ensure the same, a matchless editorial board was set up. Every individual on the board went through rigorous rounds of assessment to prove their worth. After which they invested a large part of their time researching and compiling the most relevant data for our readers.

The editorial board has been involved in producing this book since its inception. They have spent rigorous hours researching and exploring the diverse topics which have resulted in the successful publishing of this book. They have passed on their knowledge of decades through this book. To expedite this challenging task, the publisher supported the team at every step. A small team of assistant editors was also appointed to further simplify the editing procedure and attain best results for the readers.

Apart from the editorial board, the designing team has also invested a significant amount of their time in understanding the subject and creating the most relevant covers. They scrutinized every image to scout for the most suitable representation of the subject and create an appropriate cover for the book.

The publishing team has been an ardent support to the editorial, designing and production team. Their endless efforts to recruit the best for this project, has resulted in the accomplishment of this book. They are a veteran in the field of academics and their pool of knowledge is as vast as their experience in printing. Their expertise and guidance has proved useful at every step. Their uncompromising quality standards have made this book an exceptional effort. Their encouragement from time to time has been an inspiration for everyone.

The publisher and the editorial board hope that this book will prove to be a valuable piece of knowledge for students, practitioners and scholars across the globe.

Index